"Dr. Janowitz has created a plan for success. With years of experience, intense education in personal coaching, and a physician for 20 years treating tens of thousands of patients, his insight into developing a **personal plan for health and success** is all within the pages of *The Synergy Health Solution*."

—Dr. Elliott Grusky DC, FICC
Author and Professor of Clinical Chiropractic Pediatrics
Miami Hurricanes Team Physician, 1993–2018

"Dr. Janowitz's understanding of **total health and wellness** is why I love his practice as well as his teachings. You can feel this every time you are around him and throughout the pages of his book."

—Justin Dailey
Lead Pastor, Action Church

"Dr. Eric Janowitz has been an instrumental leader in the healthcare community of greater Orlando and has positively affected thousands of patients. *The Synergy Health Solution* describes his **whole-person approach to healthcare** for the reader and emphasizes his preventative methods to wellness. Dr. Janowitz provides an easy-to-implement outline for readers into becoming **healthier versions of themselves**."

—Dr. Todd Sontag, DO
Primary Care Physician, Orlando Health

"*The Synergy Health Solution* enables us to re-think some of the fundamental, yet often-neglected, aspects of life. Dr. Janowitz's perspective is refreshing. It reorients the reader toward **health and prosperity** and provides a **concrete roadmap** to do so. If the same rules are understood and applied to business operations, the impact could be significant on the firm's culture and bottom line."

—Ze Wang
Associate Professor of Marketing, University of Central Florida

"Dr. Eric has long been **a champion of healthy and well-balanced lifestyles** for his patients and community. It is exciting how so many more people can now similarly benefit from Dr. Eric's gift for motivation and the wisdom he shares in *The Synergy Health Solution*."

—John Woodson
Registered Patent Attorney
Allen, Dyer, Doppelt & Gilchrist, PA

"*The Synergy Health Solution* is a fine example of the exceptional **compassion** that Dr. Janowitz has for his patients and the community. Full of actionable advice, I highly recommend this book."

—Dr. John Barnett, AP
Acupuncture Physician, Orlando Acupuncture

"It is with great pleasure and admiration that I fully endorse *The Synergy Health Solution* written by my colleague and dear friend, Dr. Eric Janowitz. I am convinced that future readers of this artful masterpiece will be given the additional **motivation and knowledge** they need to live healthier lives."

—Dr. G. A. Lopez
Professor of Medicine, University of Central Florida

"Dr. Eric Janowitz looks at **health in a completely new and innovative way** in *The Synergy Health Solution*. Health is more than calorie counting, more than obsessing about a certain image. Dr. Janowitz teaches us that health is about living to your fullest potential in all aspects of life. I am certain that thousands upon thousands of people are going to walk away from reading this book with a **renewed perspective on health**, the realization that is within full reach, and a clear roadmap on how to attain it."

—Alyssa Chandler
Life.Church Copywriter

"*The Synergy Health Solution* is a **superb compilation of health and goal directed advice** on how to live one's life. As a neurosurgeon, I plan to personally implement many of the topics Dr Janowitz covers!"

—Nizam Razack, MD
Neurosurgeon, Spine & Brain Neurosurgery Center

"Dr. Eric Janowitz laid out a **life's manual** with invaluable insights for anyone who wants success in health and life, regardless of what you do or how gritty your goals are."

—Lincoln Salmon
Entrepreneur, Insurance Agent, and Coach

THE
SYNERGY
HEALTH
SOLUTION

THE ULTIMATE FRAMEWORK TO UNLOCK YOUR HEALTH POTENTIAL

DR. ERIC JANOWITZ

ISBN: 978-1-7345767-0-2 (paperback)
ISBN: 978-1-7345767-1-9 (hardback)
ISBN: 978-1-7345767-2-6 (eBook)

This book is dedicated to …

my supportive and encouraging parents,

my best friend and wife, Dawn,

my gifts from God—Asher, Journey, and Jesse,

my mentor and dear friend, Dr. Elliott Grusky,

and all the patients I have been blessed to serve—

you all inspire me to bring out my greatness.

Alone we can do so little; together we can do so much.

—Helen Keller

CONTENTS

Section 1: The Inner Work

Quadrant 1 Power and Quadrant 2 Purpose

Section 2: The Outer Expression

Quadrant 3 People and Quadrant 4 Process

CHAPTER 1

WELCOME TO THE FRAMEWORK FOR ACHIEVING YOUR OPTIMAL HEALTH

Welcome to the Synergy Life! This book is designed to transform the way you think about getting results in your health and, ultimately, in your life. Life is meant to be lived. Life is meant to pursue meaningful work and contribution. Life is meant to be enjoyed. You are here for a purpose, and the world desires the best version of you. It is my intention to help you squeeze all the juice out of your experience in this world.

The Synergy Health Solution is about two things: your health and how to maximize it. Following the rules of general society is not going to help you achieve great health. Society and technology have created great advancements, but now people are too accustomed to quick fixes involving little time and effort. Access to information, products, and services are so easily obtained that people are losing their emotional muscle to endure what it takes to obtain lasting health. Society now promotes convenience and comfort over real health transformation. Let's face it, it's an easy sell. If a product can make us feel good *now* and give us temporary comfort, our busy and tired society will buy it. However, staying in your comfort zone will never help you achieve your greatness.

What to focus on? Who to listen to? Why do you want good health? What is the vision for your health? How about the vision of health for the people you are responsible for? What steps should you do to protect and enhance not only your health, but the health of those important to you? As leaders in our own family or our corporate family, these are the questions that confound us and ultimately get us stuck. They can immobilize us while every day our life passes by and our health and the health of the ones we care for diminishes further.

The Synergy Health Solution provides an overarching framework so you can handle all these questions, dilemmas, and much more. We all need to take a leadership role in our own health. As heads of families or leaders of organizations, we need to guide our people so they grow to reach their best lives as well. This book will serve as a personal coach to guide those willing to assume a leadership role in their health on one of the most important journeys in life. See, without your health and the health of those people important in your life, you and they cannot be great, I mean, really outstanding in ALL areas of life. Healthy people, families, communities, and organizations can accomplish so much more when we become even better together. Creating outstanding health is possible.

The "Possibility Doctor"— That's What They Call Me

I am a doctor who has served around twenty thousand patients, seeing a new patient every hour in my chiropractic practice since it opened about 20 years ago. I am writing this book based on decades of experience helping people get well. I see my patients as amazing people who have actively played a role in helping themselves achieve their best. How? Rather than sitting on the sidelines and witnessing their health decline, they took action when they came to see me. I am both grateful and inspired by them. Many patients have been dealing with years of chronic pain or other health issues. They also come to me with the limiting belief that their *current* health condition is their *permanent* health state for the rest of their lives and that they simply have to learn to deal with it. This limiting belief is one supported by our current health system that generally conditions us to believe that a lowered state of health is expected because "we're just getting old." Instead, I have helped patients see what is possible for their lives by removing the obstacles stopping them from fully expressing their health. Because I believe so greatly in my patients and their ability to improve their health and their lives, they've come to call me the "Possibility Doctor," a title I'm proud of and stand by.

I am a coach. In my desire to help fully understand the nature of what patients are going through and discover better ways to guide them through their health journeys, I attended professional coach training. The coaching model works not only in sports, but also in all areas of life, including and especially in health. In *The Synergy Health Solution* I use a coaching model to help you bring out your greatness.

I am a professional speaker. I have been speaking to audiences about health and performance issues for the past 20 years. Helping people explore their health in a group setting and communicating to them on both the intellectual and emotional levels has helped me reach more people than the one-on-one interactions of my daily patient care. Simply put, this message is too important. These concepts are far too great. And time is way too precious for me to limit my communication to only one person at a time.

Hence, the reason for writing this book.

This book will expose you to the guiding principles that shaped the quality of my life. These principles took years for me to develop and to uncover, and they are principles I derived from a number of different sources—university degrees, seminars, books, great people in my life, professional coaches and consultants, and lots of reflective time. Now that I have you hopeful and excited about diving into *The Synergy Health Solution*, let me give you some early insights into the concepts that we will be discussing in this book.

Synergy

What is synergy? After lecturing on this concept to thousands of people, I've come to discover that very few people really understand and actually appreciate the concept of synergy. Simply, most fail to see the profound effect synergy can have on their life.

Imagine if the math education you had in elementary school stopped after you learned addition and subtraction.

$$50 + 50 = 100$$

Not too difficult math, right? There are certainly more math techniques that exist beyond simple addition and subtraction. Yet, this is how people tend to live their life and, in particular, their health.

Using this limited technique, we go through life saying:

- *If only I can take away some calories* [subtract], *I will be healthy.*

- *If only I add this particular food or supplement* [addition], *I will be healthy.*

4

This thought process goes even deeper:

- *If only I owned the* _____ [insert the shiny object of the moment], *I would be happier.*

It can even be:

- *If only I had this* _____ [relationship, career, or health issue gone, financial problem solved], *then life would be happier.*

Addition and subtraction = boring and limited.

When you really take a step back, you will see that many people often sustain and settle for lives of simple addition and subtraction.

But, what if one day you woke up, and things were different? What if, all of a sudden, you were shown new math—a new way of thinking? Imagine how life would be different if you lived by multiplication and division. Using the same 50 and 50 numbers, we now get:

$$50 \times 50 = 2,500$$

Simply adapting a new technique to our number 50, we created 25 times greater return on our outcome! This is synergy in action. Synergy is about multiplying the results in your life by combining things in such a way that the results don't simply add up, but rather they multiply. Imagine the state of your health where your efforts at improving it are multiplied. With such an improved state of health imagine how revitalized your experience of life as a whole would be!

Applying this book's synergistic framework will procure these high-octane results for your health, which, in turn, will grant you an invigorated whole life experience. After all, once the state of your health vastly increases, you can't help but enjoy everything you do each day even more. From waking in the morning, to collaborating with your team in the workplace, it will all simply be more engaging and rewarding when you're in a state of greater vitality.

Put addition and subtraction *to rest* in your health. Insert multiplication *to the rest* of your health … and life.

Synergy is about combining things in life to produce results that are greater than the sum of the individual parts. Living a Synergy Life is possible. As already mentioned, people have called me the "Possibility Doctor," and I am going to outline this synergy-based framework for optimizing your health to show you what great possibilities it offers you. You are already doing it in parts of your life without conscious knowledge. I bet we can find synergy in action in the areas of your life where you are producing positive results and experiencing a high degree of satisfaction. Randomly, it is already happening, and you are reaping the rewards. The difference is once you put this book's framework intentionally in place, it ensures more of your life multiplies and bears exponential fruit.

The Synergy Success Cycle Framework

What *The Synergy Health Solution* offers is a framework—the Synergy Success Cycle—to ensure that you address all the major areas used for restoring, optimizing—via the multiplying effect of synergy—and protecting your unique health needs in a manner that's methodical, cohesive, and thorough.

The Synergy Success Cycle focuses on four quadrants, called the "4 Ps"—power, purpose, people, and process—to show you how to develop a deeper, inspiring, and personal health plan to create a sustainable and ever-evolving approach to optimizing your health. The Synergy Success Cycle and its four quadrants are particularly effective because of their synergistic approach to optimizing your health. When you set into motion the cycle's "4 Ps," the multiplying effect that results allows you to make exponentially greater gains in your health than if you worked on a few areas of your health separately.

I want to acknowledge that each of the four "4 Ps"—power, purpose, people, and process—could be a book on its own. That is how deep the concepts go. However, what is even more necessary than inspecting at length each of these topics individually is a global framework for optimizing your health. What's crucial is the big picture plan with its designated elements working in concert, feeding into each other to build upon and influence each other, to reap beneficial multiplying effects with each revolution of the cycle. That's what matters. The Synergy Success Cycle removes the random, sporadic, and isolated approach that so many people take in attempt to better their health. It replaces it with a perpetuating system that through its moving parts doesn't simply allow a positive gain, but rather a magnified positive gain. That's the synergy effect.

Admittedly, the individual quadrants of the Synergy Success Cycle are not new. However, it is the complete framework and its specific sequence that is original and highly effective. *The Synergy Health Solution* will be life-changing for you and your health. It has been for me.

Not Ideal or Ideal—Where Do You Fit?

One way of determining if *The Synergy Health Solution* is the right book for you is for me to describe who this book is *not* right for. If any of the following describes you, then I do *not* recommend you read this book:

- *People who are not willing to take responsibility and a leadership role to protect and enhance their own and their people's health.* Health is not going to happen to us, but rather it is a gift given to us that we must work on enhancing and protecting actively. This means that you are going to have to do the work!
- *People who want a quick-fix.* All quick-fix solutions to our health—for example, simply taking a particular drug or nutritional supplement, or getting a certain surgery—are not going to impact our health overall for the long term. Feeling good temporarily is nice, but living a long, healthy, happy, and productive life feels much better and allows us to reach our full life potential.
- *People who are unwilling to take the time to learn a holistic, integrated process to regain their health.* Individuals or leaders who will not invest the time and energy to discover and examine the four quadrants of the Synergy Success Cycle and take the time and effort to implement the steps.
- *People who just want specific, "cookie cutter" health tips that offer short-cuts but are not specific to their own health or that of the people in their organization.* This book is a framework to help you customize and reach your and your team's unique best health. Simply offering a one-size-fits-all approach will not work or be personally satisfying or sustainable in the long run. You will, however, be able to discover through this process your best approach to reaching your goals, and you'll be able to guide your team to do the same.

Now that you understand who this book does not suit, let's look at characteristics of the ideal reader. If any of these describe you, then you will find this book incredibly interesting and you'll greatly benefit from it:

- *People who value preventive health care.* People who understand the importance of preventing health problems and are willing to take responsibility to protect it.
- *People who are dealing with a health problem.* People either who are experiencing a new health issue or who are suffering from a chronic health problem AND are willing to take responsibility to fix it.
- *People who strive to achieve and get motivated by big goals.* People who have a lot of things that they want to accomplish in life and understand that their health and the health of those who are important to them are necessary to achieve their goals. Again, as leaders, they are willing to take responsibility to enhance and preserve health for themselves, their family, their teams, and those they impact.
- *People who value having a system.* People who want a framework to create their unique best version of their health versus simple, generic health tips.

If any of the "ideal reader" characteristics describe you, welcome home. You will enjoy the journey. I expect you to bear great fruit not only in your health, but in all the lives in your circle of influence. That's what synergy is all about—being able to maximize and make your health and your life even better by getting clarity and applying the four quadrants outlined in the Synergy Success Cycle. It is my hope that you are inspired to not only apply this framework in your own life, but to also share this framework with all the people in your life—both personally and professionally.

Professional and Corporate

As I see it, professional and corporate leaders and their team members make ideal readers of this book. As those of you in the business world already know, it is critical that you and your employees take responsibility for your health in the same way that you take responsibility for your work. Letting your health go by the wayside in the pursuit of a professional life has consequences, not only for your career but also for your family, hobbies, relationships, and longevity. So those of you who are high achievers in the business world, you and your team members will benefit greatly from what this book provides. Benefits for corporate-level achievers include the following:

- The Synergy Success Cycle essentially is a global success framework that leaders can use for many applications in their company.
- This big picture vision for optimizing health supports corporate leaders to protect their own health with all the intense and burdensome responsibilities they have, as leaders.
- This framework helps team members to attach greater purpose to their professional life while at the same time promoting a mindset of responsibility around their health, which aids them to work better and smarter.
- A team that takes greater responsibility for their health by fully addressing all the components of the Synergy framework increases their chances of staying healthy, energized, and at the top of their game.
- Teaching the framework to the team creates a universal language to communicate all the areas required for success in optimizing health.
- This framework establishes more energized, engaged, and satisfied employees because it is a whole-person, whole-life framework for addressing health.

I encourage corporate leaders to read this book both with an eye to optimizing their own health, as well as the opportunity of establishing it as part of their company's culture. An exponential number of wins will result: for you, your employees, your business's bottom line, your family, employees' families, the list goes on and on.

For a Deeper Dive

This book is an incredible tool distilling decades worth of knowledge. At the same time, I recognize that people learn differently. While some people learn best when reading, others like to hear stories explaining practical applications of these principles. For those who want to continue listening to this conversation, we will be launching a **Synergy Life Podcast** where I will be interviewing the best of the best in their area of expertise. We will crack their code on how they have applied the Synergy Success Cycle in their life to create their own personal and powerful Synergy Life!

To learn more about and listen to our podcast visit www.TheSynergyLife.com.

Then there are those who have a deep burning desire to take in the concepts in a more personal way and really flush them out. These rare individuals desire to tie their intention with action! For those high achievers or for those who may be stuck in a rut, I will be launching an online university—**Synergy Life University**. Synergy Life University will offer online modules filled with actionable video lessons, led by me, with small incremental steps that will help you uncover ALL the pieces of the Synergy Success Cycle as they relate specifically to you.

The challenge is that we all like, and gravitate towards, the things we are good at. The tendency can be to focus too much time on those areas because it feels good, creates certainty, and gives us quick wins. The challenge, therefore, is that we fail to spend the necessary time, energy, and focus on our harder areas. By engaging in the **online Synergy Life University program**, you will not skip steps. You dramatically increase your chances of living your best life the more you are engaged in the process. Don't get me wrong, this book will create breakthroughs in your life *if* you read *and* apply the lessons. The question is simple—how far do you want to engage in this process? Remember, this life is not a dress rehearsal and every day counts.

To learn more about the online Synergy Life University visit www.TheSynergyLife.com

Finally, the Synergy Success Cycle framework has the capacity to transform not only individuals and families but also corporations and organizations. Teaching this framework to your corporation creates a common vocabulary and dialogue to help propel and enhance the health of your team. Any business leader who values health should consider having this material taught at their team events as part of a keynote. As I have customized this framework for organizations, I ask that if you find this information valuable, you consider the opportunity to help me enhance and inspire your team's health by sharing these principles. Such corporate talks demonstrate to team members that leadership cares not only about the bottom line, but also about the health of their team.

To learn more about the customized corporate Synergy Life workshops visit www.TheSynergyLife.com.

Seeing as this book is about optimizing your individual health, before we visit the Synergy Success Cycle, let's take a look at health itself. As I've already shared, I'm a licensed chiropractic physician who has seen around 20 thousand patients in my 20-plus years of practicing. As a result, I have a lot of experience regarding people's individual health journeys, and I have also made some observations about our healthcare—or rather, "sick care"—system. That's where we start: health over the decades, healthcare vs. sick care in America today, disease, and dis-ease.

CHAPTER 2

HEALTH, HEALING, AND DIS-EASE

You have to work harder as you age just to maintain the same health results you enjoy today.

—Dr. Elliott Grusky

The big goal of this book is to deliver a framework, the Synergy Success Cycle, that you can put to use to achieve and then maintain your optimal health. As such, health, healing, and perspectives on healthcare are necessarily at play in our journey together. In this chapter, I'm sharing my own "insider" insights on these issues, so you can better locate yourself in your optimal health journey and also realize the many choices you have in how you want to proceed. In turn, once we embark on the Synergy Success Cycle, I expect you'll be even more eager to engage with the 4 Ps to get the cycle spinning and enjoy the synergy effect you create and deserve.

Healing Over the Decades

The *"invincible twenties"*—we are a society where many live in chronic pain. Hence, the birth of the opioid crisis and the subsequent emergence of medical marijuana. Pushing through health problems and ignoring the warning signs, our bodies wear down. Sure, this pushing through or ignoring worked when we were younger. When most people are in their **twenties**, most health issues tend to go away with a good night's sleep. In our twenties, we can abuse our bodies as many did during sports activities and other lifestyle activities, including enjoying turning 21 with the new freedom of consuming alcohol (at least legally!). In our twenties, we are discovering ourselves and often are seeking intimate relationships, so there tends to be a lot of late-night socializing and drinking. In your twenties, your body is robust and can handle it.

Cracks in our health begin—in our **thirties**, most people get a glimpse of their invincibility. What took a single night's rest to recover and repair in our twenties now can take several days. A night of partying can linger a bit longer. An ache from playing a sport we loved in high school sticks around for a few more days. We are not quite as energetic as we used to be. We are trying to carve out a living for ourselves and tend to be working a lot of hours. Many of us are getting married and starting families. Others are "marrying" their career and starting their journey up the corporate ladder. And then there are people doing both! Lots of achieving and lots of doing, but our 30-year-old body is keeping up with us at a pretty good pace.

The 40-year warranty expires—enter the **forties**. This is when I believe that the "warranty" on our body expires. This is when the car with a 36 thousand-mile, three-year warranty that handled very well with little maintenance or attention starts to show signs of fatigue and breakdown. Isn't it crazy that when our lease expires is when the product begins to have issues? Our forties start to show the pain from a lack of intentional care and maintenance that was necessary, but often not crucial, up until that time. Our engine worked great for most of us through our thirties and our exterior showed only small amounts of wear and tear.

I remember the day that I turned 40. I woke up, and as if out of nowhere, my eyesight changed. The LASIK surgery that I had the week before my wedding as a 32-year-old seemed, out of nowhere, to expire. I suddenly became dependent upon glasses again. I'd thought that was a thing of the past, but no, enter the forties.

In our forties, the lingering pains or other health issues that once went away in a few days can now last for weeks or months. The forties are where a lot of patients who were active in their youth begin to seek professional help like chiropractic care. The most common phrase I, as a chiropractor, hear is, "I thought it would go away." And it did when we were in our twenties and thirties. Not so much in our forties. This is when people tell me they just take over-the-counter pain medicine. This is when I ask them how often they are doing it, and it has usually been for weeks to months at a time, not just a few days to get through the initial pain. Our forties, for most of us, tend to be the first major wake-up call that our bodies are not completely invincible.

Chronic health issues appear—enter the **fifties**. Health problems that used to last weeks or months now become chronic and part of our day-to-day lives. In our fifties and beyond, we tend to go from treating a symptom to managing a health problem. Our self-identity changes from being a person experiencing a particular symptom to being a person with a condition. We are not a person who is experiencing back pain, but rather a "back pain person." We are not a person who is temporarily heavier than our ideal weight; we now consider ourselves fat. We are not someone who is just tired temporarily; we are fatigued or exhausted.

Our definition of what is possible changes. Many people in their fifties have adopted a mindset that the activities they did when they were younger are no longer even possible. It's no longer an option. Our fifties are typically when we raise the white surrender flag to no longer experience or enjoy activities that once gave us a lot of positive emotional satisfaction. Often this white flag of surrender is a result of our health no longer being able to support our body. Our lack of health creates a lack of motivation and a lack of confidence that our body will be able to sustain those previously enjoyed activities.

You can see where this path leads throughout the decades, and it only tends to decline further through our sixties, seventies, eighties, and nineties. Each decade requires more effort and energy. I remember my chiropractic mentor telling me that a person has to work *harder* each decade to simply get the *same* return. That's a tough pill to swallow, but sadly after working with so many patients, I believe it to be true.

The health crossroad—so, what do you do? How will you respond to the information I just delivered? One option: you can throw up your hands and say, "Why bother?" But seeing as you have already identified yourself as an "ideal reader" for this book (remember—from the first chapter?), I know that's not the attitude you'll take!

Another option: you can be empowered by knowing the road ahead of you requires a higher level of intentional effort. You can determine that you have to have a plan and accept that you have to work harder than you did at earlier points in your life. This is the first step in protecting, maintaining, and enhancing your health. And because you've begun reading this book, you've already taken that first step. Congratulations.

Another important step is recognizing the flaws in our current state of healthcare (using that word lightly) and actively deciding to reclaim control of your health for yourself, your loved ones, and the people you lead.

Healthcare or Sick Care System?

For almost ten years, I have worked with the University of Central Florida—go Knights!—College of Biomedical Sciences as a guest speaker, speaking to nearly ten thousand pre-medical students who are striving to be some type of healthcare provider. Most want to be medical doctors, surgeons, neurologists, osteopaths, and pediatricians. Several are attracted to a particular health field based upon a personal health issue and the positive impression their healthcare provider made on them during their time of need (you'll soon learn that this is the case for me!). I love the fact that these students are attracted to a chosen health field, as they are significantly ahead of the curve in their professional development.

What does concern me, however, is the lack of clarity these young future doctors have regarding the true nature of health. Professors rarely help medical students understand the philosophical differences between the various health care approaches—from a traditional medical model versus a more holistic approach. Having an appreciation about these distinctions is important for the future health care provider, to ensure that their own personal "view" or philosophy of health matches how they want to deliver care and ultimately the type of doctor they want to become.

It seems that this lack of clarity has trickled into our whole healthcare system. Do Americans have a true "healthcare system"? Or is it more of a "sick care system"? Don't just take my word for it. A recent landmark report from the World Health Organization stated, "The US health system spends a higher portion of its gross domestic product than any other country but ranks 37 out of 191 countries according to its performance."[1] So, we spend more money than anyone in the world on healthcare, yet we get poor overall HEALTH results. We do, however, rank number one in emergency care. What does this all mean?

It means the focus is on trying to react to crisis as opposed to enact positive health-building practices before any symptoms occur. If you desire crisis- or symptom-based care that reacts to emergencies, then the US is where you want to be. Also, realize that managing crises is the most expensive (and painful) way to manage your health.

But, if you want to focus on really getting healthy, then our current system gets a failing grade. Besides an annual physical, when does someone typically engage with a traditional healthcare provider? During times of good health or when they are symptomatic and in some sort of crisis? Also, what does being "sick" even mean?

We will dive into this in more detail in a later chapter, but for now, let's explore some basic definitions. According to the World Health Organization, health is a "state of complete physical, mental, and social well-being, not merely the absence of disease or infirmity."[2] As you can see, this definition is far more encompassing than just merely someone having no apparent symptoms. In fact, can a person have no symptoms and yet be unhealthy? Of course! We all know someone that "appeared" healthy yet died of a sudden heart attack with little to no warning. You have also heard of someone that went for a routine check-up ,or some other tests, only to discover that they had cancer. Did the lack of initial symptoms mean they were healthy up to that event or discovery? No way, my friend.

Disease vs. Dis-Ease

Health is not an on-off switch. Someone doesn't go to bed on a Sunday healthy and wake up sick on Monday. Health is a dynamic range on a continuum where people tend to sway on a particular part of the spectrum. Their health potential on this scale does not improve without some proper attention. If health is a range from 100% to 0%, with 100% equaling perfect health, and

0% completely unhealthy and unable to sustain life (death), then somewhere around 60% and *below* would be the area labeled "dis-ease" or lack of ease or function.

Most early health problems, if not trauma-related, are really "dysfunctions" of the body versus a full-blown disease process. A disease process may show evidence in the lower ranges from the range of 59% to 1% on the health continuum. Most people struggle with some underlying health issues that have been masked, pushed through, or ignored to a point where there now exists a full-blown "diseased health state." If the test is *positive* on the report, only then does it become *real* to the patient.

The problem is that most modern diagnostic tests only have the capacity to identify certain health conditions when there has been an accumulation of damage to the body over time. In other words, they are not as sensitive to early health breakdowns of dysfunction that if left unchecked leads to a full-blown diseased state. It is in the state of *disease* on the continuum where MRI, CT scans, lab tests, or other diagnostic procedures yield positive results listed on their reports. This often transforms a person's perception of their current state of health. They now have a formal "diagnosis" describing their symptoms. The healthcare system and the person themselves now go by the label of *sick*. If it is on the report, then it is real to the patient.

As devastating as some news can be, many people who have received a formal diagnosis often feel a sense of relief, or, ironically, even a sense of victory, because they finally feel like they know their actual health problem. Perhaps they have been complaining to their doctor, spouse, coworkers, or friends for some time, and now they have a "real" problem that our sick care system can treat with an array of potentially dangerous drugs or invasive surgeries.

The truth is, when someone has enough accumulated damage to their health, where an area turns into a full-blown disease process, they are now certainly behind the eight ball.

Consider a person who feels okay overall but knows something is off or has had some lingering recurrent symptoms. They go to the doctor who runs a series of tests and they come back normal. How does the doctor communicate the "normal" results to a patient who knows they are not feeling right? How does that patient interpret and use these "normal" results? How have you handled any past result that yielded no positive test finding, but you still knew deep inside that something was wrong?

After consulting with thousands of patients over 20 years, most patients are confused by negative test results. They often hear the doctor stating that there is nothing wrong with them and they are just "stressed." The "treatment" is often some psychotropic drug like an anti-depressant or anti-anxiety medication because they are told that their condition is all in their head. This leads them down an unfortunate, expensive, chronic, and dangerous path into now being prescribed a drug that is often a "life-time drug." Of course, Big Pharma likes this. However, this could have all been prevented by understanding the healthcare continuum.

Irritable bowel syndrome lacks any confirmatory tests, but rather it is a rule-out diagnosis. A rule-out diagnosis occurs when a doctor runs a test and does not find positive results. Like a lower GI test that comes back negative for polyps, ulcers, or other pathology, yet the patient has constipation or diarrhea episodes. This is because irritable bowel syndrome is a "dys-function" and not a disease. It lies somewhere between 100% and 60% on the health continuum.

Stress tends to aggravate a person's health condition and makes them feel even more powerless. They become victims of their problem and get even more frustrated because no formal test confirmed their ongoing health issues.

Our traditional healthcare model in the US is not properly set up to interpret, handle, communicate, or care for patients with functional health problems, meaning folks that are not suffering from a diagnosed pathological condition like diabetes or cancers, but where their health is not working close to its optimal state. People with functional health issues know innately that something is off and they just don't feel right, but their traditional doctors aren't giving them any real answers. There is a growing sector of doctors called "functional medicine doctors" who are shedding more light to this area on the health continuum. Chiropractors and other alternative healthcare providers, such as acupuncturists or naturopaths, have a greater edge in understanding and caring for functional health problems compared to traditional medical doctors. These healthcare providers have a different viewpoint, which we will discuss later on in chapter 7.

As mentioned already, routinely I meet new patients that have been experiencing health problems, such as headaches, and who have resorted to taking daily over-the-counter pain medication for extended periods of time in an effort to simply feel better and get through the day. They do this because they have been to their doctor, underwent testing that was "negative", yet they continued to suffer. Only when they have an alternative physician evaluate them, are they able to get a fresh perspective and a fresh approach that often aims to correct the underlying cause of their issue.

Sadly, patients have forgotten that over-the-counter medications are so available and commonplace that they no longer think of them as chemical drugs. They fail to realize that ALL drugs have side effects and create some level of toxicity in the body. In fact, to be classified as a drug, a substance has to produce some "effects" to a person's physiology. The pharmaceutical industry simply labels the desired effect as the *reason* to take the drug and other effects as *side effects* because those are non-desired. Effects are effects. They are all *effects*, and most of the time, they do not correct the underlying dysfunction.

Common vs. Normal

This leads us to another core concept regarding your health and a huge trap preventing you from unlocking your health potential. Most patients equate what is "common" in their health as "normal." Again, daily, I question every new patient if they ever get headaches. Many will pause briefly and say no. I sense there is something there in their body language telling me otherwise, so I dig. They often tell me that they just get "normal" headaches. I ask about frequency, and they tell me as little as once a month or as often as several times a week ... or day! They often misinterpret their abnormal symptom as "normal" because it is "common" in their personal life and prevalent in society. This is far from the truth.

Heart disease is the leading cause of death in the US. It is unfortunately very common. Does that make it normal? Cancer is the second leading cause of death. Again, common, but is cancer the sign of a normal healthy person? Of course not. Diabetes was extremely uncommon until recently, where many primary doctors have one-third of their patient base being managed for it. Does the *commonness* of diabetes now make it a sign of normal optimal health? What about the skyrocketing obesity epidemic—normal optimal health or, again, common?

The problem is when you label your non-optimal health condition as "normal," two major things happen. One: you tend to push through it as part of normal life, and you become dependent on taking some form of medication to mask the worsening episodes. Two: you ultimately accept it as part of your life and who you are. You essentially live in a state of tolerance and acceptance of your intermittent symptoms, and you merely give up, surrender, and move on. I have seen this literally thousands of times.

When you live in toleration of your dis-ease, then you prevent yourself from seeing that there is a much greater health potential out there for you. Your definition of what is possible shrinks. **Your normalization of your common health problems is at the core of preventing you from reaching your optimal health potential.** Your normalization becomes your blinders to the riches that are just around the corner for you.

In my practice, I typically spend 45 minutes consulting and evaluating a new patient, face to face, as we get a real grasp on their overall health profile. You heard me right. Not a mere five minutes listening for a symptom to quickly lead me to a paper prescription pad to treat a symptom. A big part of my role as a leader for their health is to help them get an accurate assessment of where their health truly is and create a vision for where they want to take it.

In chiropractic, 99.5% of the patients we typically see do not require going to the emergency room. They are not on their death-bed. They are, however, like a dripping faucet, where each drop released becomes a lowered state of overall health. It's like what they say about boiling a frog. You place a frog into boiling water, and it will jump out immediately. But if you put it in a warm pot and slowly turn the heat up, the unaware frog will tolerate the dangerous condition and die in that boiling water later on.

We need to create personal leverage in our lives to where we do our best to avoid the "boiling water" events. We must put a stop to the "slowly heating" events that eventually erode and destroy our health and our lives. The Synergy Success Cycle we explore in this book will help take those blinders off and create the leverage you need in just the right areas you need it in.

The next chapter continues our examination of health-related insights and issues, so you have thorough information to make the best decisions for your health and the health of those whom you are leading.

CHAPTER 3

HEALTH AT ITS CORE

*If we are creating ourselves all the time, then it is
never too late to begin creating the bodies we want
instead of the ones we mistakenly assume we are
stuck with.*

—Deepak Chopra

To understand health at its core we need to look more at the
system that controls it all—the nervous system. According to *Gray's Anatomy*, a textbook of human anatomy,
the nervous system controls and coordinates all functions of the
body. The central nervous system consists of the brain and spinal
cord. The peripheral, or extended, nervous system starts from the
nerves exiting the spine and branches out to relay information to
every cell and tissue in the body. This is accomplished by a direct
connection of nerves to tissue cells or via hormones, chemicals
released as designated by the information supplied from the nervous system. The nervous system truly is the master system of the
body.

In chiropractic, it was drilled into our heads the importance of the nervous system and all the science that goes behind that. We are educated on the power of the body and its ability to heal via the nervous system. Think about it. What is the difference between your body and a cadaver? Both have the same parts and are put together and organized in a similar fashion. What is missing in that cadaver that causes the heart to no longer beat or the lungs to no longer breathe? In chiropractic, this is called "innate intelligence." Innate intelligence can be called "the spirit" by some, "Mother Nature" by others, "inborn intelligence," or even "life force." The actual name we call it means less than the appreciation that some element outside of the parts brings our body to life!

Another key concept is that the body, *your body*, is designed to heal. Think about it, if you get a cut on your hand, you do not need to fix your injured tissue consciously. No mental effort on your part rushes white blood cells to kill and defend the body against external bacteria that may have breached your skin. You do not consciously summon the body to bring clotting agents to the rescue to stop the bleeding, preventing you from potentially bleeding to death. Combining the power of both your nervous system AND your innate intelligence allows for function and true healing. Cut a cadaver, and you do not see the same reaction without innate intelligence at work. That is the difference!

As a chiropractic physician, we work with these three major principles. First, the deep appreciation of the nervous system as the master controller of the body. Second, innate intelligence that flows through our body and in particular through our nervous system. And finally, that the key is to remove the interference preventing the intelligence to heal. Chiropractors tend to find this structurally by locating and releasing an unwanted pressure on the nervous system that ultimately interferes with and prevents us from reaching our best health.

Stress, Breakdown, and Repair

Another way to understand your health potential and how to maximize it is by asking yourself this fundamental question: "In this particular area of my health, are the current stressors in my life causing my body to break down faster than it can be repaired?" Your health will continually decline, like inflation depleting your savings, if your body's ability to repair is outpaced and outnumbered by the amount, intensity, or sheer duration of the stresses you put on or into it.[3] As concluded by multiple researchers in a variety of studies: as stressors accumulate, an individuals' abilities to cope or readjust can be overtaxed, depleting their physical or psychological resources, in turn increasing the probability that illness, injury, disease, or psychological distress or disorder will follow.[4, 5, 6, 7] The stressors we described above can also affect the physical body and can cause spinal pain through neural pathways from the organs being stressed.

Physical Stressors

As you can see, both chemical and emotional stressors can produce a physical effect on the body. Obviously, direct physical stresses affect the body too. There are two categories of physical stresses on the body—macro-traumas and micro-traumas. Macro-traumas are significant isolated events or injuries that cause trauma to the body, such as a car accident, lifting injuries, sports injuries, and falls. These are often easier to identify than micro-traumas.

Micro-traumas are small, abnormal, destructive forces that over repetition and time can result in significant damage to your physical health. Just like one cheeseburger and fries at your favorite fast-food chain is not going to make you sick, years of poor food choices will rob you of your health—micro-traumas work similarly. Physical micro-traumas can result from poor sleeping positions and carrying items, such as a baby, a heavy backpack, or a heavy purse, too often on only one side of the body. Others can result from work-related stress due to prolonged sitting at a computer or standing in one place at a workstation. Smart phone technology has further worsened and weakened our posture with repetitive prolonged neck flexion. We really have to educate our children on the devastating effects of poor posture due to the technology that is such a part of their lifestyle. Our kids are raised on devices and compound that with heavy backpacks, increased school demands, and sports and you have a recipe for early arthritis and years of pain.

Again, these micro-traumas are like the frog being slowly boiled because in isolation, they don't appear to be harming us. In truth, these can often be harder to correct because you not only have to focus on correcting the damage already done to the body, you also have to retrain decades-old habitual patterns that define how you've been moving unconsciously every day.

More Than Your Genes!

As noted already in chapter 1, the goal of this book is to help you unlock your optimal health potential. Since the discovery of the human genome, science has created a lot of certainty in the minds of people that we are genetically predisposed to develop certain conditions. This has caused the public to believe we cannot change or influence our health outcomes. Essentially since the human genome project mapped out many of our genetic flaws or weaknesses, the pharmaceutical and medical device industries have been salivating. These giants of healthcare are ready to sell their chosen solution to the poor, unfortunate souls who are predisposed through their genetic flaws. If our genes were unchangeable and our fate was written at the moment of conception, then there would be no need for a book describing how to unlock your potential. The lock would have been sealed, and the keyhole glued shut.

Our genetics, in fact, have been proven to be only a single piece of the health equation through the recognition and advancement of the field of epigenetics. Epigenetics is the study of the changes in organisms caused by *modifications* of gene expression rather than alterations to the genetic code itself. In other words, our genetic code is like a loaded gun filled with bullets of potential health problems—like cancers or heart disease—but the expression (or realization of those conditions) can be modified by lifestyle choices. Our genes are only possibilities, not guaranteed eventualities.

Epigenetics is the silver lining in the doom and gloom of genetic weaknesses. As you'll soon learn, by applying the Synergy Success Cycle to your health and life, you can systematically learn how to make positive mental and emotional changes, which we're calling your "inner work." Doing this inner work will cause you to attract the right people and processes to stack the odds in your favor.

You not only should feel a sense of hope, but also appreciate that there exists a very real and powerful way to design better health and, therefore, a better you, which brings us to the Synergy Success Cycle—what you've been waiting for since the start of the book!

CHAPTER 4

THE SYNERGY CONCEPT AND THE SYNERGY SUCCESS CYCLE

Synergy - the bonus that is achieved when things work together harmoniously.

—Mark Twain

In the previous chapters, we discussed health and healing and some of the pitfalls of our current healthcare system. We also touched on an exciting field of science called epigenetics, and, more than anything else, I hope you are inspired by the fact that the quality of your health is not set in stone. It is not predetermined. You have choices on how to achieve and then maintain your optimal health. You can and should take an active role in optimizing your health by having a framework to make it possible. And that brings us to the concept of synergy and the Synergy Success Cycle, the focus of this book.

Creating the Synergy Success Cycle, which lies at the heart of *The Synergy Health Solution*, has been a work in progress through the application of principles I have discovered over my 20-year history of personal and professional development. The concept of synergy has been in my mind, heart, and spirit since I was 26 years old. The first time I learned of synergy was from one of the most powerful personal development books I've ever read—Stephen Covey's classic *The Seven Habits of Highly Effective People*. Covey's sixth habit, "Synergize," is about putting all the habits together in a way that makes the practices much more powerful.

"Synergy" is defined in the *Cambridge Dictionary* as "the combined power **of a** group **of things when they are** working **together that is** greater **than the** total power achieved **by each** working separately."

In my chiropractic practice, intentionally called *Synergy* Oviedo Chiropractic, we employ the concept of synergy in regard to our use and application of multiple therapeutic healing treatments. We combine the use of chiropractic adjustments, physical therapy, massage therapy, surgery prevention strategies like spinal decompression, and non-addictive, non-drug pain relievers like high-end tissue-healing class 4 lasers. Now all of these services can be helpful for our patients on their own. But when we properly combine them to the patient's specific health issues, the results are dramatically better than the individual therapies. That is synergy in action.

In the various areas of your life, you have processes and procedures that are often combined to produce higher results than doing each of them in isolation. For instance, a great husband and a wonderful wife by themselves, separately, can do powerful things, but when you combine them together, they can achieve truly amazing things. That's the multiplying effect of the positive synergistic model. The same can occur in the business or healthcare world, like my practice. At Synergy Oviedo Chiropractic, we use multiple doctors that, by themselves, are super, but when you combine the knowledge, experience, and skills of the physicians and place them under one roof taking care of the entire patient base, the results become phenomenal.

The first step, though, is recognizing that the concept of synergy exists. The second is going through the process of examining the various areas of your life where you can apply the multiplying power synergy affords. This book is specifically going to provide you a framework to create a synergy effect in the area of your health. I started with this first book focusing on the health aspect because it truly is the area that impacts how engaged we can be to improve ALL the areas of our life. It is impossible to really maximize the other areas of your life—career, finances, recreation, and relationships—if you don't have a solid health foundation.

Synergy: Looking at the "Math" of Life Differently

Often, doing things in combination can produce an "addition effect." In other cases, doing too many activities or the wrong activities can create a "subtraction effect" because adding unnecessary or counterproductive actions will decrease productivity and results.

Synergy, on the other hand, provides a "multiplication effect." Similar to learning math, you need to first learn how to add and subtract—adding or taking away new life activities. Then you can do more advanced math like multiplication and division where synergy comes into play. Again, synergy provides results that are greater than the simple sum of the individual parts.

The first shift that needs to occur in your mind is that you can, and you deserve to, have the synergy concept work to expand your health and life. You need to start asking yourself, "How can I add multiple activities in my life that would make exponential positive changes?" When asking that question, it is important to understand that the selection of those activities is important. That is where the Pareto principle comes into play.

Maximizing the Right Activities: The Power of Pareto Principle

The next important key concept to applying synergy in your life is the Pareto principle, nicknamed the 80/20 rule. According to the *Business Dictionary*, the Pareto principle is defined as the observation that where a large number of factors or agents contribute to a result, the majority (about 80%) of the result is due to the contributions of a minority (about 20%) of factors or agents. Investigations suggest, for example, that some 80% of the sales of a firm are generated by 20% of its customers, 80% of the inventory value is tied up in 20% of the items, and 80% of problems can be traced back to 20% of causes.

The Pareto principle essentially means that there often is an *imbalance* of input and output, which means that *certain* activities can produce greater results than others. For example, in investing, you find about 20% of stocks in your portfolio are generating higher returns and account for a majority of your gains. In working with teams at the workplace, you often find that some team members are more productive when serving on a committee than others. For me running a private chiropractic practice, about 20% of my patient base produces about 80% of the patient referrals. I should add that while the Pareto principle is nicknamed the 80/20 rule, it may not always be exactly that ratio. Regardless of the exact ratio, you need to know that the principle exists.

Creating the Synergy Health Solution in your life involves insights from both concepts: the Pareto principle and synergy. First, you need to discover your "high octane" activities—the 20% key activities, contacts, and/or resources—that will help produce your greatest results regarding achieving and maintaining your optimal health. Then you learn how to synergize these key activities in such a way that will produce dramatically more productive and fulfilling results in your health, thus in your overall life.

Speaking of your overall life, let's look into that using a construct called the Wheel of Life.

The Wheel of Life

We don't just live one-dimensional lives. We wear many hats. Globally we tend to break our lives into two categories: professional and personal. In reality, there are many more areas that create the fabric of who we are. In my professional coach training, we help clients identify areas they want to focus on or need to focus on using a powerful tool referred to as the Wheel of Life.[8] This wheel provides a visual aid to help us see the many areas of our lives.

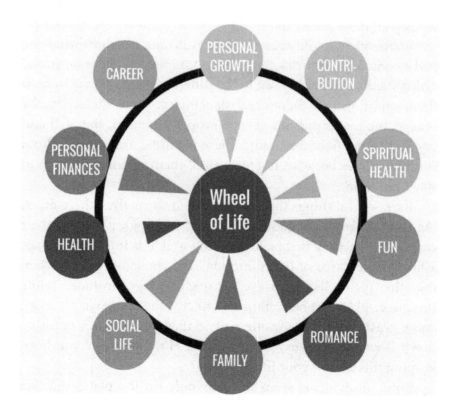

As you can see, the Wheel of Life is much more extensive than considering your life in only two major realms like most people's viewpoint: professional and personal. The Wheel of Life acknowledges that we are much more complex than that. For example, we are professionals in our chosen work. We are children of our parents. We may be spouses or parents. We manage finances and need to earn a living (or better, create financial independence.) We have friends and a deep desire for connection. We have hobbies and things we do to blow off steam (however, many seem to have forgotten how to do this in the busyness of life!). We are spiritual beings having a human experience. We have a desire to grow and a desire to contribute. It is, therefore, essential that we FIRST create a high level of health to give us the energy, drive, and ability to keep all these plates spinning.

I remember an old episode of Ed Sullivan's TV show where he had a comedian, Henrick Bothe, spinning several plates on sticks. The comedian feverishly ran to the different dishes trying to keep them spinning and, therefore, balancing on small sticks. One by one, as the plates did not get the proper attention, they fell and crashed to the floor, breaking. These life areas are just like those spinning plates because, in truth, all of them require attention to stay in motion.

I see several things that happen when we analyze these areas. One is that people are good at focusing on a single plate, like their career, and keeping that plate spinning well. It is impressive to see a finely tuned area of life in motion. The challenge occurs when the other plates, like marriage, get neglected. For instance, while the career plate can be spinning perfectly, the marriage plate can come crashing down. Another plate that often comes crashing down if we are too busy is our health. How well have you been keeping this area of your life spinning?

Some individuals seem to focus only on the plates that are crashing, and they fail to see that some plates, in fact, are doing quite well. These people often can feel depressed or have FOMO— fear of missing out. So, just as focusing on select plates that are spinning well can result in other important plates crashing down, this opposite response of focusing only on the crashing plates is not healthy either.

Here is the good news—ALL the areas, all the plates, work together in synergy. For example, when a person focuses on their health, initially they may choose to start an exercise program. Then they begin to select healthier food options. Now with some increased self-esteem and added energy, they might be more playful with their significant other, so romance kicks up a notch. Maybe now that they've created more energy reserves, they increase their connection with their children versus just crashing on the couch. In this way, I want you to see that all the areas can synergistically move us closer to achieving our best life (multiplication). But, when these areas are neglected, they can also synergistically move us farther away (division).

All the areas are significant, but as a physician who has served, listened to, and helped thousands of patients, health is the foundational area of life that needs our full attention. Without our health, we cannot have the energy, the desire, or the ability to make any real impact in this world for ourselves and the people we love and serve. The other areas simply will only be able to rise to the level of an individual's health capacity. Besides, what is the point of having massive wealth if you don't have the health to enjoy it?

This is why this first *Synergy Solution* book in the series focuses on the area of your health. All the other books on this subject should refer you to this one first, as you should not focus on the other areas in your Wheel of Life until you have this plate spinning at a solid speed.

So far, we have outlined health and its critical primary role in allowing us to live our best life. You have been exposed to the concept of synergy and how it can multiply the quality and quantity of your results. Now, we come to the point, my friend, where we can plug these concepts into a unique framework that will ensure you "hit" all the major areas of focus to create the success you desire and deserve. Like driving a high-powered electric car with tons of torque, prepare to launch your best health with the Synergy Success Cycle.

The Synergy Success Cycle: The key to unlock your potential

Think of your health potential as a giant treasure chest with four separate keys to unlock and open the case. These four keys represent the major elements, or quadrants, of the Synergy Success Cycle. To literally "unlock" your health potential, we must use the proper key that is unique to you. Like your fingerprint, the key to open your best health is unique. People can try to borrow another person's key, but it just doesn't feel right and doesn't quite allow for the same opening.

The four keys that open your treasure chest are your power, purpose, people, and processes. These "4 Ps" make up the four quadrants of the Synergy Success Cycle. In the duration of this book, we will take a deep dive into each of these 4 Ps. Let's begin with a brief overview of them.

Raising your health potential occurs when you discover how beautifully this Synergy Success Cycle works. Let's reconsider the Wheel of Life. In each of its ten areas, we have a certain potential that propels us up to a certain level of success and satisfaction or a limited potential that causes us to slip down in the other direction. In fact, my definition of human potential is the synergy of power, purpose, people, and process for each area of your life. These 4 Ps make up the four quadrants and are the critical elements of the Synergy Success Cycle.

- Quadrant 1—Power
- Quadrant 2—Purpose
- Quadrant 3—People
- Quadrant 4—Process

Quadrants 1 and 2: Inner Work

The first quadrant—power—is your perception of your own power. It is your self-identity and the confidence level you have in yourself and your ability to impact particular areas of your life. Within your power, there exists your unique gifts and talents, your values and viewpoints, your beliefs and limiting beliefs, your rules, and how you celebrate your victories. Chapters 6 to 10 are dedicated to power, the first quadrant in the Synergy Success Cycle.

Your personal power is raised or lowered by these drivers. If we perceive that our health power feels low due to current symptoms, dis-ease, or disease, then our ability to create a strong purpose will be limited, which brings us to the next quadrant.

Quadrant 2, the purpose quadrant, consists of your compelling why, your ultimate vision, your inspiring goals, and your promises. Purpose is the fuel, the energy, the spice of life. Purpose makes work meaningful and fills our spirits. Work ceases to feel like work when it is purposeful. This will be discussed in detail in chapters 11 to 13.

The level and intensity of your Power (Q1) fuels your purpose (Q2). Power (Q1) generates purpose (Q2). The level of your purpose will be limited (both raised or lowered) by your current level of power. **We can *want* to have a large, inspiring, and impactful purpose, but it will *only* rise to the level of our power, or self-confidence, in the specific life area.** For example, in our health, we can have a purpose of running a marathon or living to 100. If, however, we have internal limiting beliefs about what exercise means or what aging means, then our internal critical voice will tap our shoulder and say, "Who do you think you are fooling?"

Our level of purpose, no matter how profound, will be limited by our current sense of power—or confidence. Our creativity and internal strength to stick things out when they become tough can only rise to our level of power, which essentially creates our ceiling for the level of purpose in our lives. The emotional juice that purpose generates will slip away if our understanding and appreciation of just how powerful we are is low, which could then build momentum to set the whole cycle into effect to our detriment. You see, while we aim to use the Synergy Success Cycle to positively reinforce and impact health and life, it can also work in reverse. If we do not use our strengths, that discourages us from having a vision, which then leads us to attract or seek out others who do not value health, so that our actions tend to be those that promote poor health habits.

Conversely, by harnessing the first two quadrants in the cycle, we can reach health success. For instance, as we build confidence and our power increases, then our old less-than-ideal purposes and goals begin to feel limiting because we are different. In this way you can see how these two quadrants feed into one another to create the synergistic effect for the better or for the worse.

Celebrated author and speaker Wayne Dyer once said, "As you change the way you see the world, the world you see changes." These words apply so eloquently to the influence and impact of our identity and self-concept (thus power, Q1.) When we change our perspective and viewpoint, then the entire experience of life changes. As our perception of the world changes, almost automatically, we can adopt a more positive, more impactful self-identity. With this newly formed identity, we can see new levels of purpose (Q2) that we were once blind to.

When we are clear on all the elements of purpose, magic happens. The law of attraction brings us in proximity to people, places, events, and circumstances that match our level of thinking and intention. When we have clarity of purpose, there are parts of our brain that activate our awareness to recognize how we can accomplish our goals.

There is a special part of the brain called the reticular activating system (RAS), and it is a powerful beacon for focusing your awareness. The RAS is the body's anatomical part that ignites the Pareto principle and sparks synergy. You have probably heard the saying, "As the student is ready, the teacher appears." This means that when you are ready to grow in a particular area, suddenly, as if by magic, you meet new people in your life that can help take you to the next level. This is the people (Q3) part of the Synergy Success Cycle that is activated by your compelling purpose (Q2).

Quadrants 1 and 2, power and purpose, are called the "inner work" of the Synergy Success Cycle because they happen inside us in the mind. As the great Napoleon Hill pointed out, "Whatever the mind can conceive [purpose, Q1] and believe [power, Q2], the mind can achieve." Power and purpose are personal inner concepts that we must observe and reflect on to discover and grow.

We are more powerful than we give ourselves credit for, but we all have some internal struggles based upon past events and the stories we tell ourselves about what those events mean. Because all things start in the mind, we start the Synergy Success Cycle in the mind as well with the inner work of nurturing quadrants 1 and 2. The mind game is what we need to master first. The good news is that the greats of the past recognized this to be true to unlock our best health and life potential, so they've supplied us with lots of options for doing this inner work.

Quadrants 3 and 4: Outer Expression

Quadrant 3 of the Synergy Success Cycle is people. To introduce this quadrant let me share a recent event from my life. A patient of mine who had struggled with a painful and emotional flare up thanked me, with tears of gratitude in his eyes, for helping him become pain-free and to return to his normal life. Moved by his kind words, I told him that a purpose filled doctor needs patients to serve, just as importantly as the patient needs a doctor. The point is that we don't live life on this planet alone. As strong as we are, we need people in our life. The people quadrant, therefore, consists of our role models, mentors, and teachers, the people on our team, the people we serve, and our peer group. Chapters 14 to 16 discuss the people quadrant (Q3) in greater detail.

From the people in each area of our life, we tend to learn "best practices" on how to produce even better results. The quality of the processes (what I'll soon introduce as Q4) we utilize is in direct proportion to the quality of people in each area. This is because we tend to use similar processes as our peer group.

Sociology, the study of social interactions, has proven that we tend to behave similarly to and act like our peer group as a survival mechanism. Besides learning best practices from the people in our life, we need people to help us with all the processes we must do to bring our purpose (Q2) to life. For example, I have a great team of doctors and support staff help me perform the thousands of processes (Q4) we do each month to serve our patient base.

The fourth quadrant—process—can be broken down into the work we do on our health, the work we do in our health, and the standards we choose to execute that work. Process (Q4) will be fleshed out in detail in chapters 17 to 19. I should add that you will love the section on standards. Standards are where the gold is. Ultimately, the quality of your life is based on the quality of standards you hold for it.

Quadrants 3 and 4—people and processes—are where the rubber meets the road. It is where you get things done. People are told that knowledge is power and that is true, but having power (Q1) with no people (Q3) to influence and impact is meaningless and severely limited. Having power (Q1) and purpose (Q2) with no actions (actions = processes, Q4) to impact the world is a shame. You need to leave a positive mark on the this world. You need to incorporate the people (Q3) in your life and the systems and processes (Q4) to obtain, retain, and maximize your health potential.

Synergy in the Cycle:
Feeding Into and Building Onto

The reason it is called the Synergy Success Cycle is because all four quadrants—power, purpose, people, and process—influence one another and interconnect to create your overall wellbeing. The synergy effect that happens amongst the four quadrants has an exponentially more powerful effect on your wellbeing than each quadrant on its own or even by simply adding together the power of each quadrant.

Let's look at how interconnected and influential the four quadrants are. For example, as you learn, develop, refine, and upgrade your processes (Q4) with your people (Q3), you naturally obtain higher levels of results, success, and satisfaction. This new level of success fuels an even greater self-identity (Q1). This increased self-identity (Q1) has a synergistic effect that increases your capacity in the other areas.

With this upgraded level of power as our new baseline, our overall potential rises and expands. We can recharge and expand our purpose (Q2) to match our new internally perceived power capabilities (Q1). What once seemed impossible now seems possible, so we set our targets higher with hopefully the desire to impact a more significant number of people (Q3) on a deeper level.

This entire process of unlocking your health potential is opened up by finding your unique combination of all four elements and their respective sub-elements. This cycle is ongoing and continually serves to expand and impact all the other areas of your life.

To exemplify how interconnected and influential the four quadrants are—and to tell the story of how the Synergy Success Cycle came to be—in the next chapter I relate how my life and health have played out. In reading how power, purpose, people, and process worked together to create a combined—and multiplied—very negative effect (in my childhood) and then later a hugely positive effect, you should gain an increased understanding of the awe-inspiring synergistic power of the Synergy Success Cycle. That way, when it's your turn, I hope you'll be incredibly motivated to harness this cycle and put it to work to achieve your optimal health.

CHAPTER 5

INFLUENTIAL AND INTERCONNECTED— THE SYNERGY SUCCESS CYCLE IN OUR LIVES

It is good to have an end to journey toward; but it is the journey that matters, in the end.

—Ernest Hemingway

Your story reveals patterns. Reflecting on your personal journey is a powerful tool that is often overlooked and vastly unappreciated. Even more than just thinking about it, recording it helps you see much more about who you are and allows you to identify patterns in your personal journey. In the context of this book, when you reflect on *your* story, you'll see how the Synergy Success Cycle and its 4 Ps—power, purpose, people, and process—have been at play and continue to be at play in your life. You'll see how incredibly influential and interconnected these elements are, and how it is in your very best interest, both for your health and beyond, that you harness this framework to actively determine how the cycle plays out for you; rather than letting it happen passively, and likely to your detriment.

In this chapter, I share my story to show you the patterns at work. Specifically, I will point out how the 4 Ps have been at play in my life, so you can see how interconnected and influential the parts are—and how they are likely equally so in your life as well.

The process of examining my own story ultimately helped reveal to me the framework for the Synergy Success Cycle, which then led me to write *The Synergy Health Solution*. I tell you my story not to impress you or to say my story is more special than yours, but to give you an in-depth example of the framework of the Synergy Success Cycle at work in a single person.

In delivering my story, first I'll describe my current situation. After that, I'll give the "story behind the story," which reveals the potent interplay of the 4 Ps—power, purpose, people, and process—in my life.

My Current Situation

At the time of writing this book, I am 45 years old. I have been married to my amazing wife, Dawn, for 13 years now. She has always been smart, playful, positive, and supportive. Thankfully, we have never reached any point in our relationship where we ever wanted out. In our 13 years together, we have honestly never had any major fights or major disagreements. We always have been able to support each other when the issue at hand was a "big deal" for the other. In terms of the people quadrant (Q3), I patiently waited until I found the right person to marry at the age of 32. I could have married at an earlier age, but my life would not be at the level it is today. Dawn is my best friend and my life partner.

We have a son named Asher Jayden, who is ten, and a daughter, Journey Joy, who is three. We recently brought Jesse Elliott into this world, and his smile burns in my heart. I call him "Mr. Giggles" because he smiles and giggles with everyone he engages with. It's hard for people to explain to others who don't have children exactly the love you have in your heart for them. It is like another part of the heart cracks open, and there is a new area, a new reserve, flowing with love for your children.

We live in a nice comfortable home in our community where the children feel safe to play and enjoy the outdoors. My wife, who worked in my practice and helped grow it with me for 10 years, 3 years ago made the decision to home-school Asher and play a highly active role in his and our other children's development. I founded my private chiropractic practice 18 years ago, and we have established it to the point where we do not need to take on any debt.

I hit my personal financial goal of becoming financially stable by age 30. I created that stability by living what some would say was an imbalanced life, but I was highly focused on my purpose (Q2) in helping transform the health of my community. I made a conscious decision back then to hold off on any intimate relationships and live way below my means, so I could focus on my chiropractic passion, purpose, and mission. Delayed gratification was my code of living. At that time, I focused solely on serving others, and their health results were my main areas of personal and professional satisfaction. As I progressed professionally, I was able to incorporate and expand the other areas of my wheel of life. Although, I think no one is ever fully ready to have a family, I intentionally waited until other areas in my life were in order to create a solid foundation.

I have a clear vision (Q4) for the next chapter in my life. I want to teach these legacy and generational principles that I am outlining in this book not only to my children and future grandchildren, but I have a burning desire to inspire others, particularly those in the corporate world, to start discovering and carving out their purpose in life, starting with their health. My goal is that these Synergy Solution concepts will have a multiplying effect in the lives they touch in such a way that it positively impacts the world in a significant way.

Currently, my practice has served around twenty thousand people in my community, and I have personally provided over 250 thousand chiropractic adjustments to positively impact the health of my patients. My career has provided me with tremendous personal satisfaction and fulfillment, meeting many of my needs for creativity, emotional and spiritual connection, certainty, variety, leadership, finances, and personal and professional development.

My health is strong, as is the health of my family. I have a personal trainer who comes to my home at 4:50 am, so I can "turn on" my physiology for optimum performance. I receive chiropractic adjustments regularly to reduce the physical and emotional demands that running a business and general life create. My wife selects vegan meals for us, and I consume mostly a plant-based diet with only occasional meat and dairy.

We attend a great church where the pastor is young, healthy, vibrant, and an amazing teacher. He is a master at telling us what we need to hear but not always want to hear. He goes for leadership over being liked, and that is what I admire about him. We pray before our work at my chiropractic office, and that helps keep me centered.

From the outside, my life looks pretty darn amazing, and the truth is that most of the time, it feels that way too. However, it is far too frequent that when you look only at someone else's success, you fail to see the depths of their personal journey and how they got there.

There is a popular image on the internet that describes the "iceberg illusion."[9] It demonstrates that people only tend to see and judge the success of others by what they see on the surface, "the tip of the iceberg." This surface includes the individual's success, victories, and accomplishments. However, what most of us don't see is all the work that it took for the person to create those accomplishments over years. This includes the persistence, failure, sacrifice, disappointment, discipline, hard work, and dedication. That's what makes up the bulk of the iceberg that's hidden below the surface of the water.

Similar to the iceberg image, we only tend to see the "tip" of a person's iceberg without realizing all the other efforts and obstacles in a person's journey that lie below the surface. It is typically in this "submerged" part of a person's story that the significant elements of the Synergy Success Cycle—power, purpose, people, and process—have been at work to bring them to their current situation. And that brings us to the "story behind the story" of my life.

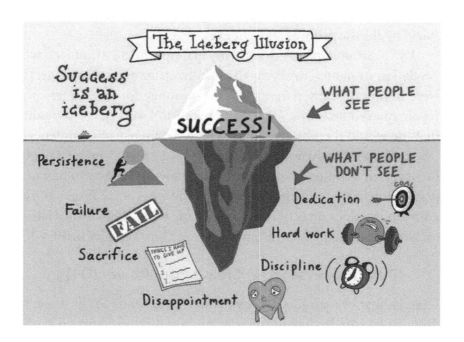

My Synergy Journey

As a six-year-old child in elementary school, I was a skinny little boy living in the suburbs of Miami, Florida. I felt powerless (remember, power lies in quadrant one and determines whether and how much our synergy cycle turns to create positive gains and success), shy, and intimidated by my peers. Why? Because I suffered from a severe "lazy eye." I recall systematically avoiding eye contact with others in my futile attempt to hide my eye condition. I recall every time I talked to someone they would turn around or to the side, trying to see if I was talking to them or someone else because my "lazy eye" drifted elsewhere. I couldn't control my eyes, so I felt out of control when I communicated with my peers. I felt deeply disconnected.

If the eyes are the window to the soul, I felt that my soul was shut off from the world. I had given up on even trying to connect with others. Isolation and weakness were my emotional home, my identity (Q1). The condition of strabismus itself is called "cross-eyed," or even worse, "lazy eye." How powerful is it to be "cross" or "lazy"? All I wanted was straight eyes.

I begged and pleaded with my parents to do whatever we needed to straighten my eyes. Thankfully, at age eight, my requests were honored as my parents saved up money for the surgery to repair my crossed eyes. Well, the operation "worked"! I thought that life would then be amazing! With a new sense of confidence, I began interacting more with the world. I created new friends, focusing on building relationships with new students who had no prior knowledge of my past "lazy eye," my weakness. Things were going in the right direction, at least for my eyes. That is, until later on when I learned what the surgical procedure actually involved.

Poor Processes (Q4) Create Poor Power (Q1)

Here is how eye surgery works to "fix" strabismus or "lazy eye." The eye essentially has muscles at the top, bottom, and on both sides that control the eye's movement. For a crossed eye, there is an imbalance in the muscles on the sides. The "normal" functioning muscle on one side wins the tug of war competition and pulls the eye toward its direction because the opposite "weak" muscle cannot counteract it. The surgery is designed to cut the normal muscle to make it as weak as the weak muscle!

Parents reading this: imagine if the doctor told you that they were going to "fix" your child by weakening them. In other words, making them as weak as their weakest link! No one would sign up for that. It's ridiculous and absurd, but that is what they did to me.

Many times, in life, we can be so committed to the outcome that we fail to take the time to understand the philosophy behind the process and the implications that the process can create. You see, if you weaken one area of your health, it does not occur in isolation. Other areas inevitably weakened too.

Now fast-forward about a year, I developed a scoliosis in my spine. Scoliosis is a twisting and rotation of the spine that not only affects your physical appearance, but it also affects the nerves exiting the spine that travel to all the muscles and organs in your body. Scoliosis causes muscle and overall energy fatigue because muscles that are normally at rest are "firing" and using more of the body's energy. It leads to areas of chronic spasm and tightness, often leading to decreased chest expansion and, therefore, less-than-optimal breathing patterns and capabilities. The ribs are constricted in their motion, which leads to a sub-optimal oxygen intake. The imbalance in the spine also causes abnormal pressure on the bones, joint, and discs. Scoliosis leads to accelerated arthritis, joint pain, pinching of nerves, and negative effects on the many nerves that are meant to feed vital energy and information to the body. The abnormal stress on the discs can lead to disc bulges and herniations often causing not only back pain, neck pain, or headaches, but also pain, weakness, or numbness in the arms or legs.

Here's what I believe happened to me: the muscles that control the eyes are impacted similarly in the brain as the muscles that control and influence the spine. They are both core and central in the body. When my eye muscles were essentially further weakened and rebalanced artificially by the surgery, that weakness spread to my spinal muscles, causing imbalances that led to scoliosis. So now one problem incorrectly handled led to another problem. In this way, we can see the negative, undesirable synergistic cyclic effect at play in my health, with one unwise health decision feeding into and encouraging another even greater weakness.

Amazing People (Q3) and Updated Processes (Q4)

I now was confronted with a new obstacle. Do I undergo another surgery, this time on my spine to "correct" my crooked spine by inserting two metal rods in my back and having them literally bolted to my developing spine in order to keep me upright? Or do I find another solution?

Thank God my dad had back pain. This caused him to seek a chiropractor by the name of Dr. Elliott Grusky. Dr. Elliott sat down with me and my dad and said that there was a choice. Essentially, I could have the surgery, which would straighten my back very quickly by having rods put in, or undergo long-term chiropractic care to optimally correct and stabilize my spine.

The problem with "straightening" the spine with rods is that the rods, then, essentially rob the muscles from doing their work to grow and stay strong. Have you ever broke an arm or a leg and had it in a cast? How did the muscles look afterward? Nice, thick, developed, and strong? Or smaller and weaker? If you don't use it, you lose it. They will atrophy and weaken. This is what would happen with my spine, and back too, with the rods.

This correcting of my spine with metal rods felt a lot like the process of "fixing" my eyes by cutting the normal muscles to weaken them to the level of the weak muscles. I would have ultimately had a straighter but weaker spine. So, with this new education and a doctor who provided me an alternative process, I pursued the path of correcting my spine through chiropractic care and exercises to strengthen the weaknesses. It was not a quick fix, but most quick fixes do not last in the long term.

This shift in treatment choice only occurred when new people (Q3) came into my life, people like Dr. Elliott who showed me an alternative, more empowering approach (process, Q4). I went from a low personal power (Q1) of just wanting to be fixed regardless of consequence (lowering to the level of a weak link) to a strategy of strengthening my weakness and rising to new levels (a higher sense of personal potential, power, and control of my situation, Q1 and Q2).

Looking back, this was a critical tipping point in not only my health but also my personal development. My synergy cycle that had been turning and propagating ever-negative outcomes was suddenly moving in a new direction, one that was offering positive elements, elements that once they built momentum would multiply (via synergy) to produce massively positive results in all four quadrants.

The decision to seek care from Dr. Elliott Grusky, in my opinion, was the biggest, most powerful catalyst in my life. Not only was Dr. Elliott a highly skilled pediatric chiropractor, he had this radiant energy and this sense of power, love, and certainty. He still has this way about him 40 years later. Every time I was adjusted by him, not only did my physical body feel better, my soul was nourished. The way he spoke to me instilled a sense of worth and value that I got nowhere else outside my home. Blessed, my parents were very loving and encouraging, but I felt they had to be because they were my parents. Dr. Elliott was the only person outside my home to give me energy and confidence.

Dr. Elliott has made such an impact on me that we named our youngest son Jesse Elliott Janowitz. The name Jesse is from the bible. Jesse was the father of King David and means "gift from God." We intentionally and lovingly named our son Jesse Elliott because Dr. Elliott was truly a gift from God in my own life.

Stronger Purpose (Q2) Increased Belief in My Potential

Next, I recall being in one of Dr. Elliot's treatment rooms when everything clicked and the lights went on in my mind.

Dr. Elliot asked me, "Why do you get a fever?"

I was about nine years old, so I answered simply, "Because you are sick." He educated me that the body creates a fever when there is a bacterial infection. The bacteria cannot survive the higher temperature, so the fever kills them, and then the body's temperature returns to normal.

He then asked me, "So why would you want to take medicine to artificially stop the fever?" I responded that it didn't make sense, and he agreed.

Then he asked, "Why do you cough?"

Again, as a young child, my response was "Because you are sick." He then explained that typically there is something in the lungs, and coughing is the body's natural way of getting it out. So, he asked me, "Why would you want to take a medicine to stop the cough?" I realized that taking the medicine did not make sense, and he agreed again.

Dr. Elliott further explained that the difference between chiropractic and traditional medicine is that traditional medicine is typically focused on treating the symptom while chiropractic is about improving the function of the body. He showed me the following nerve chart:[10]

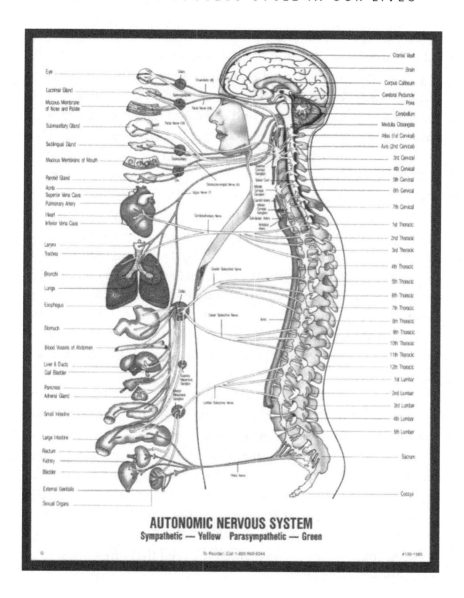

AUTONOMIC NERVOUS SYSTEM
Sympathetic — Yellow   Parasympathetic — Green

He explained that the way the body works is that the brain controls the body. It does that by sending nerve messages down the spine and out to all the muscles and organs in the body. He traced the chart showing me that each nerve exiting the spine

55

controlled specific muscles and organs including the lungs, stom-ach, and heart. At that time, I was into science experiments involv-ing electricity where I used batteries connected by wire clips to dimmer switches. He added that when there is good alignment to the spine, the nerves are free and clear, and the power going to all parts of the body is healthy and strong. But when the spine is out of alignment, it causes the nerves to be interfered with and essen-tially shuts the power down to those specific muscles or organs "like a dimmer switch."

My eyes and heart were opened that day, and my mind was lit up. The person who filled me with positive energy while helping me strengthen my weakness taught me two compelling princi-ples. Those principles impacted the course of my life. One was the power of questions, which we will dive deep into later. And the other was the principle of chiropractic about the removal of nerve interference to allow the body to express life versus the common practice of Western medicine: treatment of symptoms. My life was forever changed.

Now I learned these powerful principles, but I was on the passive receiving end. Later on, while under his care, Dr. Elliott saw my interest in all the science behind chiropractic care. Instead of just completing my treatment and moving to the next room, like many doctors unfortunately do, he stopped and recognized my interest. He sat me down one day and encouraged me. By this point, I was feeling a bit stronger emotionally about myself (Q1) because I was taking an active role in helping myself get stronger (Q4). At that young age, he planted the seed that I may want to be a chiropractor myself (Q2).

My Purpose (Q2) Tipping Point

I now had a shift in purpose (Q2). My early-life purpose was to not be seen and to hide behind my "lazy eye." My second upgraded purpose was to strengthen my weakness in my spine and take control of my health. Both were focused on me. This new third transformational purpose was the idea of helping others improve their health by correcting *their* spines and nervous systems. This transformational shift in purpose I have labeled the "purpose tipping point."

I define the "purpose tipping point" as when you make a conscious, intentional shift from your purpose being solely about yourself and just surviving, to a transformational shift where your purpose is centered around impacting others and the world. You simply become the vessel for change in the world.

The Right People (Q3) and Better Processes (Q4)

A few years later, Dr. Elliott allowed me to be the first-ever student in Dade County, Florida to do an "executive internship" in my senior year of high school at a chiropractor's office. I went to classes in the morning and then interned at his office in the afternoons. I would either help in the rehab room, assisting his team with physical therapy equipment, or I would assist in the administration with filing.

My favorite activity though was going room to room with Dr. Elliott and witnessing him adjust his patients. While making notes as he called out to me what he was doing, I also observed how he interacted with all his patients. This man gave positive energy and inspiration not only to me but everyone he touched! I keenly watched how he expertly adjusted patients. The way he talked them through the procedure. I was in full observation mode, seeing not only the technical aspects, but also feeling the energy he created in the room. It was magical and exhilarating.

So, I went from no awareness to awareness of alterative healing strategies. I then moved to proof through observation by watching a blackbelt perform his craft. But seeing something performed and doing the same thing are two entirely different levels of the game of mastery. I then went on to the University of Florida, where I took all my pre-med classes in addition to earning a degree in psychology. Looking back, I knew Dr. Elliott had a special way about him, but I wanted to quantify and study it. Studying psychology seemed a natural fit.

I then went to Logan College of Chiropractic in St. Louis, Missouri. This was an easy decision because Dr. Elliott had gone there, and I had a cousin who happened to live minutes from the college with a basement where I could live for free. It all fell into place. Entering with a competitive edge by already knowing that I wanted to be a chiropractor since age nine, having a mentor, and already having interned in an amazing office during high school were foundational to my success.

Although I knew, I could not do. Yet.

I started a bilateral education. One aspect focused on how to pass tests with mostly As, and the second focused on how to apply the information I was learning in my future practice. You see, most people make the mistake of only focusing on the short-term. Most students pick a standard they are after (for me, that was getting the A) and only concentrate on the test itself but not the applied training the knowledge was teaching.

Since I had already had the backdrop of "seeing" my future in action by working in Dr. Elliott's office, I could "file" the new knowledge gained in chiropractic college within my mind. I studied with the intent to understand where the school education applied in my ultimate practice vision. Unfortunately, this is a massive hole in the traditional education system. Our education system needs to do a better job in helping students see the value of the new information AND its future application to fulfill their mission and life's work. That, of course, would mean that the student had some concept of their purpose (Q2), which is why the Synergy Success Cycle is so important!

The Bigger the Vision, The Better the People (Q3) You Attract

To further enhance my learning curve of practical application, I was blessed to discover a professional chiropractic fraternity, Pi Kappa Chi. I was fortunate to get to surround myself with smart, driven, and focused fraternity brothers who were farther along in their studies than I. They further helped shift my focus beyond the next exam in front of me and, instead, to the big picture. I regularly reminded myself that I was not in chiropractic college to be a professional test taker, but to be a world-class chiropractor.

The fraternity provided a unique environment where you could be a first-year student and learn from the experience of upperclassmen who were farther along with their training. As a fraternity pledge, we would be required to come to campus an hour early, before any other students arrived, and our upper-class brothers would help us develop our chiropractic technique skills. Looking back, not only did it help us, the younger students, it reinforced the upperclassmen's confidence in developing their craft too. Additionally, several former fraternity graduates would visit and share stories about how it was in the real world of early practice. I heard the highlights and challenges they were experiencing in the next stage of what would soon be my career too. What a gift!

I learned there were two essential skills to master (processes, Q4). The first was the technical skills of the craft of adjusting the spine. The second was communication. In fact, the person who taught chiropractic philosophy, Dr. "Reverend Roy," stated in our first semester that the number one determinate of your success in chiropractic is your ability to communicate chiropractic. Although, to my surprise, most of my classmates did not recall that sage advice in our senior year, I listened and consistently applied that pearl of wisdom, which has contributed greatly to my present-day success.

Actually, I now believe that principle to be much grander. **I believe that the number one determinant to success in life is your ability to communicate.** And besides communicating with others, you need to learn how best to communicate with yourself in your own personal psychology. I talk much more about this in the book when we examine the power quadrant (Q1).

The older fraternity brothers also shared personal development principles and introduced me to my early teachers: Tony Robbins, Brian Tracy, Ken Blanchard, Jack Canfield, and Mark Victor Hansen. Also, there were other great influential and inspiring doctors in the chiropractic profession that provided healthy motivation to doctors who wanted to make a big impact. I would regularly go to the public library to check out cassette tapes and next CDs. My CD player was always broadcasting people filling my brain with principles for success. I literally drowned myself in the teaching of success principles and processes (Q4).

I owe it to my fraternity brothers (Q3) for showing me that this world of knowledge and people (Q3) existed. Again, you see how the people (Q3) you surround yourself with expose you to new and innovative processes (Q4). Their messages sparked hope in me, ignited by passion, and ultimately my desire to create this work I am sharing with you.

Applying My Updated Synergy Success Cycle to the Next Chapter of Life

I made it through all the college classes over nine academic years, studying for thousands of hours and taking hundreds of tests.

My driving aim was to eventually be the "Tony Robbins of Chiropractic." When I graduated at the age of 25, it was time to start practicing.

While waiting for my national and Florida board results to grant me an active license to practice, I visited close to 50 offices in several states trying to find the most powerful (Q1) doctors (Q3) to work for and further mentor me. I sought out offices that matched my clear vision (Q2) and used protocols (Q4) that aligned with my style of patient approach and care.

I took my first chiropractic job as an associate for an amazing, hardworking chiropractor, Dr. Fogarty. I respect this man so much because he had an unbelievable work ethic and was a hard guy to keep up with. I hated it and loved it at the same time because he constantly pushed me out of my comfort zone. I created the opportunity to work as an associate in one of his practices, plus the possibility of purchasing his practice down the road. A win-win.

I then had to make another critical professional decision. Should I buy the practice and continue his vision of private practice, or stay the course and continue towards my vision and open my own practice? I drafted a 60-page business plan and met with the Small Business Development Center advisors. I lived frugally in an effort to save start-up cash reserves for a business loan. I had to work hard to avoid the "shiny object" syndrome and not buy things simply because I was now a hard-working doctor and "deserved it" (a seriously hard process, Q4, at times).

I visited other potential surrounding towns, outside of my current practice and my non-compete agreement, to find a town that I could grow with. I envisioned people saying 30 years from then, "Oh, Dr. Eric, he's been here forever." I found the town of Oviedo, Florida, and made it my own. I picked Oviedo because I knew it would be a great place to live, work, and play while raising a family. Mind you, I did not even have a girlfriend at that time, but I was always looking ahead. I found the location, negotiated my lease, selected my contractors … All was contingent on my SBA business loan being approved.

My loan was approved, and my life course was set in a new motion. But it was approved on September 11, 2001, the day America was attacked brutally on our own soil and the country was filled with fear, anger, and uncertainty. At that moment with my loan just approved, I was required to quit my job, the one that had stable success, the one that had the then current Synergy Success Cycle running in a predictably solid manner and with a predictable income. The day America was attacked, I instantly became a quarter-million dollars in debt and had to start from zero again with an empty patient base in a new town and no paycheck. All the while everyone was immobilized emotionally as they focused on the uncertainty of that time.

I could have begged my leasing agent to reverse the lease. I could have crawled back to my old employer, asking him to reverse the 90-day notice I'd had to give him. Yes, you read that right, not two weeks, 90 days, which he wanted me to do since I was still producing at record numbers for his company.

Here's why I tell you this. My purpose (Q2) was tested big time here. This was a test for me between my level of certainty of my ability to start a business from ground zero (my power, Q1) versus the uncertainty of the world that was created by that horrible day of terrorist attacks on US soil. Thank God I had been planting the seed of wanting to be a chiropractor since age nine! That decision to open a new business in uncertain times was fueled by the momentum of purpose (Q2) and the level of personal power (Q1) I'd created over the prior 18 years. The people (Q3) in my life reinforced my decision that I could do it.

One year after the practice opened, we went from zero patient visits per week to over 500. The average chiropractor sees 100 patients per week, to give you an idea of how a giant purpose (Q1) fuels growth. I decided that in order to grow my practice and meet the patients where they were, I rented a kiosk at the local mall. Every day that first year of my practice, I was either at the office treating patients, or I was at the mall meeting potentially new patients. I had to fight the internal battle of looking strange by being a doctor who was in the middle of the mall on weekends when everyone was enjoying their time with their family. How was I viewed as a doctor sitting at the mall? Very few doctors in the country were doing this method of connecting with their community to find those in need. At times it was fearful, discouraging, demeaning, and disheartening.

But my fear and doubts were squashed by my beliefs (power, Q1). I was more committed to my goal (purpose, Q2) of creating a successful practice that helped thousands of people compared to my fear of not looking good or appearing abnormal. And through the disciplines of community outreach, high quality patient care, and financial rigorousness, I was able to pay off my 30-year student loan debt in just 18 months after starting my own practice. At the same time, I also paid off my seven-year business loan debt in a mere six months.

Staying and Straying from the Course

Your purpose is going to be challenged throughout your life, especially the bigger your purpose becomes. In business and life, you also have to fight temptations that affect the core of your philosophy and standards to handle negative impacts. Florida had legislative changes that were negative to the chiropractic profession. Without chiropractic having a large lobbying impact, insurance companies and other major healthcare provider types can be much more powerful in getting what they want (power, Q1, obviously works for organizations as well as individuals!).

At that time, in an effort to innovate, survive, and meet the changing demands of patient care, I decided to create a practice that would "integrate" both chiropractic and medical care under one roof. It seemed like a solid workable concept (and others were doing it successfully), but for me it was a disaster.

If I was only financially motivated, it could have worked. But I was deeply grounded in the chiropractic principles and philosophy in both care and approach. How could I practice in my main business where we believe that the body has the capacity to heal without excessive dependence on drugs, and on the other side, my medical team was prescribing drugs and doing invasive procedures? I'd made my chiropractic practice successful by being incredibly focused on caring for my patients and creating a service experience that matched top hotels. I had trouble finding a medical team that really grasped our philosophical approach and service standard. I had to lower my standard of patient experience because I needed them to make this combined model work. The medical team were great people, but they just were not great for my practice style. Consequently, at that time I felt handcuffed emotionally, financially, and philosophically.

Two years later and over a quarter-million dollars lost, sleepless nights, and a lot of heartache, I decided to pull the plug. Thank God I did because I was reaching the point where I wanted to give up. Giving up on something that I loved and wanted to do since I was age nine would have been emotionally devastating.

At that time, I kept seeing the Mercedes Benz advertising campaign that said, "The best or nothing." My practice was magical when it was purely focused on our purpose. Re-inspired, I then reversed course and returned to my original model of practice, sticking to what we did best. We solely focused on providing the best corrective chiropractic care to families. Each year after we made that decision, the practice grew. We helped more people by delivering focused chiropractic, had more fun, and were more profitable. Rather than having a medical team within our practice, we created relationships with incredible medical practices in the area that could deliver what they did best. Our patients now had access to both models of care, and we didn't have to make sacrifices in our standards.

What did I learn? Lots of lessons, including going back to your purpose (Q2). Often, we have to be threatened with the loss of something to see just how much we love something. I was in love with my life's work again.

Student Becomes Teacher

There is no way that formal educational programs like law school, dental school, medical school, or even chiropractic school can train you to run a successful business. Their job is to equip you to be competent providers in a particular field but not competent owners or managers of these services. So, after working with professional business coaches for over 15 years, it became apparent that I should learn to hone in on that skill even more. Rather than pursuing an executive MBA, I sought to become a certified professional coach. This training equipped me with the confidence and skills to not only coach my patients better on ways to help them achieve better health, but it offered me greater skills to coach my team and it spread to my acting as a professional coach to other high-producing executives in the fields of healthcare, law, and finance.

An Even Higher Purpose (Q2)

Providing chiropractic care and impacting a community is necessary and important work for me. It does, however, still come with limits. As a practice, we can only impact a finite number of patients who live or work nearby. Recently, I've had a nagging feeling inside, telling me that again, not only is the message greater than the messenger, but I must spread the message beyond my office in Oviedo. I need to teach these concepts to the world. I need to write this book, create a podcast, online university, and share this message in the corporate world despite being very comfortable at the level of my practice and the busy family life that a marriage and three young children creates. I have to push my expansion into my greater purpose (Q2).

I hope that through the story of my own life, you can see how the Synergy Success Cycle is ever-moving. How one quadrant feeds into another and another and another, so that we regularly return to the quadrants to grow ourselves in their capacities. The danger is ignoring the ever-moving cycle and allowing complacency or distraction in. Especially in regard to our health, it is vital to avoid becoming complacent or distracted.

You see, our health is our most precious asset. Without its full expression, we cannot live out the full capacity of the life we were meant to manifest. Not only will this book provide specific strategies on how to regain or retain your health, more importantly, it will also teach you a way of thinking. A way of formulating many different concepts, like recognizing and embracing your power (Q1), identifying your purpose (Q2), engaging with the right people (Q3), and doing the right things (i.e., processes, Q3) in a way that expands your health potential. All of this brings us to you. It is your turn to engage with the Synergy Success Cycle, starting with quadrant 1—power, so you can establish the framework for achieving your optimal health.

QUADRANT 1 POWER AND QUADRANT 2 PURPOSE

We start our examination of the Synergy Success Cycle with quadrants 1 and 2, power and purpose, both of which are at play actively, or passively, inside of you. As you'll see, whether you decide to harness your power with intention or let it happen by default, both ways feed into your recognition and harnessing of your purpose (Q2). Because your power and purpose happen inside you, I am calling them your "inner work." Your stance and engagement with your inner work directly correlates to the people (Q3) and processes (Q4) that you have on the outside of your life. Thus, all aspects of the Synergy Success Cycle are influencing one another, are interconnected, and can work together to create an awesome life and robust health for you—or they can create the opposite: a difficult life and poor health. And it all starts with your inner work, starting with your awareness of and engagement with your power (Q1).

Quadrant 1—Power

So that you can recognize and activate to your advantage all aspects of your power, chapters 6 to 10 examine the depth and variety that your power manifests itself. In these chapters, you'll be looking at your power in these terms:

- Chapter 6: your power in terms of your unique gifts and talents
- Chapter 7: your power in terms of your values and viewpoints
- Chapter 8: your power in terms of your beliefs and limiting beliefs
- Chapter 9: your power in terms of your rules
- Chapter 10: your power in terms of your victories and celebrations

When you realize and enhance your power in these areas of your being, you place yourself in the driver's seat for putting into motion your Synergy Success Cycle so that the other quadrants—purpose, people, and process—will be equally proactive and optimized. In turn, you establish an incredibly strong framework so that your health is optimized as well.

CHAPTER 6

Q1 POWER—UNIQUE GIFTS AND TALENTS

Your talent is God's gift to you. What you do with it is your gift back to God.

—Leo Buscaglia

Life is hard enough as it is. I believe that there is no need to add additional stress to your life if you don't have to. That is not to say that all stress should be eliminated. Think about it—you cannot increase the strength of a muscle by not applying some level of stress to it. To grow yourself in a certain area of life—for example, in public speaking, learning a new language, or expanding your group of friends—it is necessary to increase pressure in that area and add a bit more to your plate.

That being said, it is far less stressful when you play towards your strengths. When we use our strengths and apply them to our health, the path towards achieving our best health becomes easier, sustainable, and more fulfilling. Let's turn to an example: dieting. Very few people like to diet. The word even has the word "die" in it! Dieting or restricting things that give us pleasure is hard and often unsustainable in the long run. But, what if on our path to creating health, we modified our eating style or incorporated new fun activities in a way we enjoyed and that came easily to us? What if becoming healthier was more pleasurable than painful? When you recognize, appreciate, and integrate your own unique powerful strengths and gear them toward getting healthy, you will stack more wins in the health column. The more wins you have, the healthier you will become, and this will reinforce your personal health power.

Taking the time to investigate your strengths is a worthwhile investment of time and energy, not only in increasing your health, but in all the areas on the wheel of your life. After you recognize your strengths, it is important to ask yourself, "How can I further use my strength or talent to become even more healthy?" or "How can I use my personal unique strengths to become healthier and enjoy the process?" When you move beyond the purpose tipping point (again that is when your purpose is greater than just meeting your needs but rather the needs of others or major causes), you can ask, "How can I use my talents to increase my health, support those around me, and be able to better fulfill my life's purpose?"

You need to be healthy to accomplish great things in this world and so does your team—be it your family or your colleagues or employees at the workplace. Creating a life of positive significance requires robust health to make it through all the highs and lows that are going to come your way. Using your talents to become even more healthy is necessary to reveal your power not only to others, but to yourself. Again, your level of purpose (Q2) will only rise to the level of power (Q2) that you recognize and have identified within yourself.

To discover your unique strengths and talents in terms of bettering your health and even beyond I recommend the following:

- **Look to your childhood to see early formations of your strengths.**

Were you an athlete growing up? Were their particular sports or recreational activities you previously enjoyed? What hobbies or other activities did you enjoy and naturally gravitate towards? When you look back at those activities, what was it about them that made you enjoy them? Was it the physical fitness, the competition, the break from school, or the connection with other teammates? What skills were you proud of or came easily to you? Reflecting on this time in your life will reveal patterns.

- **Next, look at what you naturally like doing.**

What are the things that you do or activities that you get lost in where you are not concerned about time? Where time, you, and the activity flow without much extra drive or attention needed? These moments are often referred to as a "flow state." We have all had them. My ten-year-old son causes so much pushback on certain aspects of his home-school study, but he can get lost on the iPad building cities when playing Minecraft. He is in flow. He can play with Legos and put together complex models often without the instructions, by simply looking at the pictures. He is in flow. When any contractors come to our home to repair or build something, he follows them around and asks them a million questions to figure it out. He seeks to understand how it works. He is in flow. Ask yourself—when you are in these moments of flow, what is it about you that makes it easy to stay involved and create success? This is one way to see your natural talents.

- **Another way to get clarity on your strengths is to ask people around you.**

Ask something along the lines of "In the area of _____ , what do you think I am good at and why would you say that?" Others' insights can help reveal strengths you have that you were not even aware of. We are often blind and unknowing of our own strengths because, by their very nature, they come easy to us. We mistakenly assume that everyone has them. It is much easier to notice our deficiencies because we tend to see them through our mishaps. Too often, we focus on what we are bad at and events where the outcome did not match our expectations.

- **Finally, another way to understand our strengths is to take an assessment.**

One of my favorite ones is Strength Finders, an online assessment that offers a companion book as well. This body of work involved evaluating a large number of people (in the millions) to create an assessment tool that in only about 20 minutes provides you a list of your top strengths. The power of this work is that it breaks down 34 strengths into clear, definable terms and frames them in a very positive way. Most have an idea of what their strengths are but lack the vocabulary to appreciate them clearly and articulate them to themselves and others.

Whenever I am caring for a patient, and they are going to a job interview, I encourage them to take this test as it will help in the interview process. So far, everyone that has followed my instructions got job offers!

Part of knowing your strengths is also identifying and appreciating your behavioral style. A simple and powerful tool is the DISC profile.[11] DISC is an anacronym for four primary behavioral styles: dominance, influencing, steady, and conscientious. Here is an example of DISC:[12]

There are entire books written just on the DISC profile. Dr. Tony Alessandra, who certified me as a DISC instructor, wrote

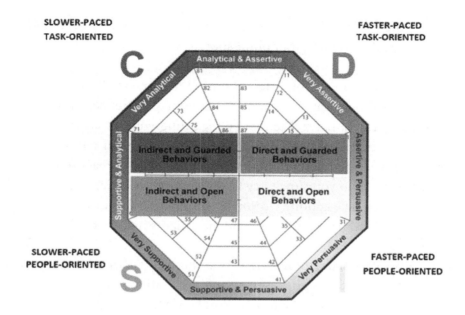

a great book on this subject called *The Platinum Rule*. You can read his book to go deeper in this area, but there are a few basic concepts that you can start to apply:

- D stands for "dominance" or director. This is a person whose behavioral talent is fast-paced and task-oriented. They get pleasure in getting things done quickly.
- I is for "influence" or socializer. This person is the life of the party whose behavioral talent is fast-paced and people-oriented. They know everyone and can be very entertaining.
- S stands for "steady." This person's behavioral talent is slow-paced and people-oriented. They excel at being supportive and making sure everyone is involved. They are sensitive to the needs of the people around them.
- C stands for "compliant." This person has a talent for being slow-paced and task-oriented. They ensure in a very

methodical and deliberate way that nothing is missed and excel at pointing out blind spots.

Your DISC behavioral style is not set in stone at all times. You are not a robot that simply reacts to your preferences. You do, however, have a natural tendency regarding your behavioral talent, and it is either D, I, S, or C. You can discover your natural talent at times when you are under stress and have to react quickly. Under stress, do you slowly try to understand the problem, or are you quick to take action? Do you go straight to tasks or confide in people? We all have a natural tendency that is not good or bad, it is just us.

A healthy behavioral style is one that can adapt and change. There are times, though, based upon the situation, relationship, or event where you adapt your behavioral style to effectively navigate through life. However, if that behavioral style is significantly different than how you best and most naturally operate, it will create stress, fatigue, and subsequent illness in your life. Be who you are. Adapt to situational and relational needs, but make sure you are putting yourself in situations where your natural behavioral style can shine more often. Make sure to have health strategies in place if you find yourself in roles where you have to veer from your natural style for a prolonged time.

In using the principles of *The Synergy Health Solution*, it is helpful to see where you specifically are engaging your natural talents towards improving your health. People tend to be either fast-paced or slow-paced in their health approach. Fast-paced people may seek foods that are already prepared, so they may frequently eat out or order in. Slow-paced individuals may find joy in researching recipes, carefully selecting ingredients at the grocery store, and cooking meals from scratch. In fitness, fast-paced people might most enjoy high intensity, fast-moving workouts like group cardio classes. Slower-paced people might focus on slow, deliberate exercises like yoga, barre, or meditation. Both extremes can invigorate someone emotionally and physically, yet their approach is entirely different. It depends where you are on the DISC profile. Seeing what activities you enjoy and that come easily to you gives you a better idea of your behavioral tendencies and strengths. If you find a particular health activity is not resonating with you, then it may be the wrong pace, so try another activity with a different pace and see how you feel.

People also tend to be either task-oriented or people-oriented. My wife can work out for 90 minutes with a DVD video by herself at home. She loves it and can grind it out. That does not work for me. I enjoy working with my personal trainer, Dane. I get massive value for not only the accountability, precision, and feedback, but also the relationship. I am not one of those types of people who love exercise, but if put in the right context for me, which for me includes being around people, I enjoy it and can do it consistently and produce results.

Task-oriented individuals can get lost when researching foods, using exercise equipment, or while reading books on optimizing health (like this one!). They may enjoy the task of preparing and cooking the meal while a people-oriented person may get pleasure in cooking with others or the thought of preparing a meal for loved ones. The point is to identify your own strengths and talents and put those to work for you to optimize your health.

Again, the fastest and often most accurate way to understand and appreciate behavioral styles is to take an assessment. I became a certified DISC trainer and have made the assessments available to my readers. Be sure, though, when answering the questions, to think about your behaviors as it relates to the HEALTH area of your life. That will give you more relevant information on helping you unlock your health potential.

To take the DISC online assessment visit www.TheSynergyLife.com and look under the resources tab.

Synergy Action Steps

1. When it comes to health, what are your strengths and talents? For example: researching, organizing, particular sports, commitment, consistency, cardio, weights, diet, communicating, supporting others, etc.
2. Where do you feel your natural behavioral tendency is on the DISC profile?
3. Ask three people, who you feel really know you, what they consider your top three strengths.
4. How can you apply the strengths they identify in you towards improving your health?
5. Have you taken any assessments like the ones listed in this chapter to gain more clarity on your strengths and talents?

CHAPTER 7

Q1 POWER—VALUES AND VIEWPOINT

Peace of mind comes when your life is in harmony with true principles and values and in no other way.

—Stephen Covey

Understanding Your Global and Targeted Values

There is a lot of discussions these days about value. The term itself has many meanings. According to *Merriam-Webster Dictionary*, some definitions of "value" include:

1. "The monetary worth of something."
This is an interesting definition because you often hear that health is priceless, and you can't put a price on it. Yet, many people's actions in how they spend their money and what they allocate towards their health are not consistent with that statement.

2. "A fair return or equivalent in goods, services, or money for something exchanged."
In health, this could be exchanging your money or insurance benefits for treatment with a physician. This could be exchanging funds for a gym membership or buying healthy foods.

3. "Relative worth, utility, or importance."
What has been the relative worth of your recent experiences with your healthcare providers? How much utility are they providing to your longevity and vitality? What about the gym you belong to but have not visited in some time? Or the food in your grocery basket?

4. "Something (such as a principle or quality) intrinsically valuable or desirable."
This definition is where we are going to spend our focus, as this one most applies to our concept.

Interestingly, *Business Dictionary* defines "values" as "important and lasting beliefs or ideals shared by the members of a culture about what is good or bad and desirable or undesirable. Values have a major influence on a person's behavior and attitude. They serve as broad guidelines in all situations." Even though this definition is specific to business, if you thought of your health as a department of your life, this may be the most relevant definition.
So, values encompass the following:

1. Important to YOU and the members of your culture (i.e., the people quadrant of the Synergy Success Cycle)
2. Desirable
3. Influencing behavior
4. Influencing attitude
5. Lasting beliefs or ideals
6. Broad guidelines that when something happens in this

area of your life, values serve as your internal judge. They "ring the bell," letting you know that a behavior is either good or bad for you.

Peaks and Valleys

We often get clarity of our values when we experience the highs and lows of results in an area of our life, called peak and valley experiences. When we experience a peak positive that creates a powerful emotional response, we should pay attention and reflect. Through reflecting on these positive experiences, we can ask ourselves why we were moved so emotionally. What about it aligned so beautifully with who we are? We can discover not only our strengths but also our values.

During powerful negative valley experiences, we can reflect on what about it rubbed us the wrong way. What about it conflicted with who we are or who we are seeking to become? Use these moments to truly clarify what you value. The same goes with frustrations in your life. Frustrations can lead to breakdowns or breakthroughs. They can provide a great breakthrough in value clarification.

Global and Targeted Values

There are two categories of values: global values and targeted values. **Global values** are ones that apply to all the areas of our life. These are more ideals that we want to see in ourselves and the world around us. Some examples include:[13]

- Authenticity
- Achievement
- Adventure
- Authority
- Autonomy

- Balance
- Beauty
- Boldness
- Compassion
- Challenge
- Community
- Competency
- Contribution
- Creativity
- Curiosity
- Determination
- Fairness
- Faith
- Fame
- Friendships
- Fun
- Growth
- Happiness
- Honesty
- Humor
- Influence
- Inner Harmony
- Justice
- Kindness
- Knowledge
- Leadership
- Learning
- Love
- Loyalty
- Openness
- Optimism
- Peace
- Pleasure

- Poise
- Popularity
- Recognition
- Religion
- Reputation
- Respect
- Responsibility
- Security
- Self-Respect
- Service
- Stability
- Success
- Trustworthiness
- Wisdom

It is not a bad idea to circle the top ten that really resonate globally with you and then narrow it down to the top five out of that list. This can help you further narrow it down when you look at targeted values.

Targeted values are values that apply towards a specific area in the Wheel of Life. Because health is the topic of this book, we should consider targeted values in the specific area of your health.

I'll add that in my practice, we take the time to understand the values of our patients when seeking to improve their health. With thousands of patients interviewed, here are some common health-related values my patients have shared, a list we'll call the Targeted Health Values List.

TARGETED HEALTH VALUES LIST
Comfort/Pain Relief

The vast majority of people, by the time they reach 40 years old, are dealing with some type of recurrent musculoskeletal pain that comes and goes. Their lack of comfort can often affect their mood, motivation, and focus. Severe pain can consume so much of a person's attention that it becomes their entire life story. Those people's lives consist of different doctor visits, managing a briefcase of pills, and conversations with friends and family that always lead to talking about their poor health and limitations. Not a fun place to be.

Function

Others value being able to do and enjoy things. Function allows you the capacity to perform the demands of your day-to-day work, such as sitting in front of a computer all day, long commutes in the car, or lots of standing or physical work. For others, valuing function means being able to enjoy time with their children, going to theme parks, playing sports, or enjoying hobbies. Function can also be enjoying greater intimacy with their spouse.

Flexibility/Mobility

The ability to move freely within themselves and around their environment.

Freedom/Independence

Freedom is not having your health limit you in any way; it doesn't prevent you from doing the things you want to do, when you want to do them, and how you want to do them. Great health provides a lot of freedom to choose how we want to live life. By contrast, think of people who have neglected their health during their "productive and providing years." They grind so hard that when they do retire (or are forced to retire due to neglected health capacity), they are not able to enjoy the very fruits of their labor, such as traveling, doing hobbies, or participating in gentle sports. Look at the various senior centers: they are labeled independent living, assisted living, and memory care. What is your ideal vision of where you want to live in your last years? What steps are you doing now to create that?

Stress Reduction

Finding a healthy way to reduce stress can positively impact your health. You get what you focus on. So, if you experience a lot of emotional stress in your life, you may want to consider how much you truly value the reduction of it.

Sleep

Sleep is essential to repair the body. Remember in chapter 3, I spoke of the major health formula. The key to health is to make sure that your body is repairing at a rate that is either keeping up or exceeding the rate of breakdown. Sleep is a critical component of resetting your physiology. Sadly, most patients rate their sleep as average or poor. The first key here is to define what about your sleep is poor. Is it trouble falling asleep, waking up throughout the night, not allocating enough time, or not waking up rested? Next, identify the causative factors, including an active mind, the environment, or tossing and turning due to pain. After that, use the framework outlined in the Synergy Success Cycle to find the right people and processes to help your unique situation.

Energy

On a scale of one to ten, with ten being the most, how would you rate your energy? If the number is lower than you like, how long has it been that way? How much do you value high energy? Where are you gaining your energy? Does your energy come from within your physiology or externally derived from a soda can or coffee cup? What is robbing you of your energy? What are you missing out on because of your lowered energy? Again, you will only focus on solving the energy equation once you place a high value on your energy.

Cosmetic

People feel better when they look their best. There are entire industries built around helping us look and present better to the world. I realize that there are some negative beliefs out there that try to create the perception that basing value on looks is superficial. The truth is that health often looks good to the human eye. When I studied pathology, or the study of disease, whenever they showed pictures of diseased tissue, the images naturally induced an internal negative gut feeling. The tissue simply did not look healthy. You can tell if a piece of meat does not look good at the grocery store. Something looks off. There are sociological experiments that demonstrate that not only our survival, but also our ability to thrive can be impacted by our physical appearance. Studies, don't kill the messenger here, have shown that people are perceived as smarter or can earn more income when they are viewed as visually more attractive.

Posture

Specific to structural health and chiropractic, your posture is a significant component to the health of your nervous system. Poor posture places abnormal gravitational stresses on the ligaments, joints, discs, and nerves in your body, which leads to pain, poor mobility, and lowered health. We all have a family member or a friend that has poor posture and walks around with slouched shoulders, forward head posture, or a hump on their upper back. Those people are not beaming with energy and are often in pain along with other health issues due to chronic nerve stress. Your posture also influences your emotional states, so having a strong upright posture exudes confidence and energy!

Longevity

Others value living a long, happy, healthy life. When I tell patients in my practice that when they turn 100, they get free care at my office, many patients emphatically state that they do not want to live to be 100. They think of being 100 as existing in an abysmal, handicapped health state. But what if you can live a long life with vibrant, strong health? My dad is 80, and I admire the fact that he plays golf almost every day!

Legacy

What kind of mark do you want to leave on this world? How do you want your friends and family to remember you? What principles, ideas, values, or contributions do people think about when they hear your name? When they reflect back on your life, how would they say you managed your area of health?

HEALTH PREFERENCES LIST

You also have health preferences you value, as described below:

Preventative vs. Reactive Care

An ounce of prevention is worth more than a pound of cure. That is true if you value health prevention. Most people wait until they're in a crisis and react to their health breakdown. There is so much going on in day-to-day life that when we are not in a crisis, most do not focus on their health but rather on their daily demands.

To make matters worse, our healthcare system favors a reactionary, sick care model because there is a lot of money to be made treating disease. If you owned a pharmacy company, would you want your patients to take your product never, only for a short, defined period of time, or for life?

Realize that if you value prevention, you have to work even harder to keep it a priority because the default societal norm is more about immediate gratification, "live for today," and pay for it later. The problem is that paying for it later may equate to chronic poor health management.

On a scale of one to ten, with ten being the most, how much do you value health prevention? On a scale of one to ten, how much is your current strategy and resource allocation consistent with your value of health prevention?

Natural vs. Artificial Health Approaches

Do you value using more natural remedies to help restore balance in your health, or do you favor more artificial, scientific, human-made approaches, like the latest medication? Both have benefits at certain stages, but do you try natural remedies first?

Conservative vs. Aggressive Care

Do you value trying conservative care first before trying more aggressive methods? When communicating to your doctors, do you make it a point to tell them that you want to try the most conservative approaches first because they have the least amount of side effects, or do you put a greater value on relief of symptoms, which could result in you taking a powerful drug with a potential for a powerful side effect?

Correction of Cause vs. Treatment of Symptoms

Same principle here as above. Do you value investing the time and energy to research, both on your own and with your doctors, the cause of your health problems? Or has your health declined so badly that all you can think about is relieving your symptoms?

Take another look at the Targeted Health Values List and the Health Preferences List. What are your top values on each list? Get clear as to why they are essential to you. Are there others that are not listed that you value as relates to your health?

Understand that these values will dictate, direct, and influence your decisions on your health and ultimately, the results you achieve. Your targeted and global values will significantly impact the level of your purpose.

Your Health Viewpoint

A viewpoint that many successful people adhere to is the concept of personal control. This is a viewpoint (and really a belief) that an individual can impact their life outcomes by their actions. If a person feels they cannot control or impact events—or have power—then they will never really ascend up the Synergy Success Cycle. In order to be an agent of change, we must adopt a belief and viewpoint that we can impact the change. If someone feels out of control, then they cannot create a higher level of purpose.[14,15] And of course, this can be easily applied to your viewpoint on your ability to be an agent of change regarding your health.

How you view health will shape your health status. The "lens" you look through in regards to your health with affect the interpretations you make when health issues occur, the actions you will take, and ultimately the results you achieve. There are two major health viewpoints: mechanistic and vitalistic.

The global mindset of the mechanistic or reductionistic point of view on health is that we are a bunch of moving parts that can be broken down. These parts or systems can be analyzed against acceptable norms—often created and influenced by the drug companies having influence over the research. The mechanistic view is that symptoms are a sign that something is wrong. The aim of treatment is designed at stopping or reversing the symptom, often with little regard to the usefulness of the symptom or the impact to the rest of the body.

By contrast, the vitalistic point of view—the one taught to me early in life by Dr. Elliott and later professionally in chiropractic college—emphasizes that we are much more than just our parts. All of our organ systems are interconnected by our nervous system, and there is an innate intelligence within each living being that provides it life. Health is more about the full expression of all the dimensions of our life—mind, body, and spirit. The body uses this intelligence and varies its approach depending on the unique situation that is occurring. This means that sometimes the body may cough to expel something from the lungs, send pain signals to help us avoid further damage by loading an injured joint or tissue, or raise our body temperature to become uninhabitable by a foreign invader. For some, fever can be considered an expression of optimal health; for others, it can be called a symptom that needs to be treated. Would you be healthier if you had a bacterial-type infection, and your body did not elevate its temperature? What about if you had something growing in your lungs, yet you did not cough to expel it? What if symptoms are the very treatment our body needs?

Take the time to reflect on these two viewpoints—mechanistic and vitalistic—and determine which one you value more. Next, determine how consistent your current health actions compare to your viewpoint and values.

Synergy Action Steps

1. What are your top five global values?
2. What are your top five health-targeted values or preferences?
3. Which health viewpoint do you connect with most—the mechanistic or vitalistic viewpoint?
4. Is your current health approach consistent with your values and viewpoint?
5. What adjustments do you need to take to be more aligned with your values and viewpoint?

CHAPTER 8

Q1 POWER—BELIEFS AND LIMITING BELIEFS

The outer conditions of a person's life will always be found to reflect their inner beliefs.

—James Allen

I n the last chapter, we broke down values and viewpoints, so you could better determine how your particular values and viewpoint impact your health. Hopefully, you gained more clarity on your viewpoint preference and your general and targeted health values. Part of the definition of values given earlier included "important and lasting beliefs." Beliefs have a critical role in shaping our human potential.

What is a belief? Looking again at the *Merriam-Webster Dictionary*, we find that a belief is:

1. "A state or habit of mind in which trust or confidence is placed in some person or thing."

2. "Something that is accepted, considered to be true, or held as an opinion: something believed."

3. "Conviction of the truth of some statement or the reality of some being or phenomenon, especially when based on examination of evidence."

Our beliefs create a feeling of certainty about what something is or means. Our beliefs form at an early age when our minds are often immature. Beliefs make the world appear less chaotic and ground us, especially during hard times. We tend to think about beliefs more in the context of religious beliefs; however, we have beliefs in all areas of our life, including our health.

In order to become the orchestrator of your life and create your best health and life ever, you need to bring to the surface your beliefs about health and the origins of those beliefs.

Again, because beliefs create your accepted standards and habits, consider the following questions:

1. What is your belief about our current healthcare system? Do you put a lot of confidence in it? Does it provide you the resources to help you maximize your health?

2. What is your belief about medication? Should it be used never, only during a crisis, or all the time without question?

3. What is your belief about where health comes from? Does it come from within, or does it come from an outside agent, like a doctor, drug, or procedure? Or does your belief about healing incorporate your faith?

4. What are some of your beliefs around yourself and exercise?

5. What about your beliefs around yourself and eating right?

Since a belief provides a feeling of certainty for how something should be, this means that beliefs inherently are limiting. Working with a set of limited concepts regarding how something "should be" often limits you to other possibilities. For instance, if you have a belief that weight loss can only occur by skipping lots of meals, then you could be blind to other avenues for losing weight.

Limiting beliefs are, therefore, false or incomplete beliefs that a person learns often by making an incorrect conclusion about something. We create limiting beliefs due to references in our lives from third party knowledge, for example, our parents, our school system, our friends, and plain old experiences. There are several categories of limiting beliefs, and we will look at four of them: generalities, false interpretations, assumptions from the past, and deep-seated beliefs.

Limiting Beliefs: Generalities

Generalities about a concept, group, or thing are a type of limiting belief. As a shortcut to handling so much information coming at us, we often make global generalities about things. For example: all thin people are ..., all super fit people are ..., and all forms of exercise are .... Generalities box you in and keep you from growing and expanding, both in terms of increasing your options for improving your health and bettering your life as a whole.

Limiting Beliefs: False Interpretations

False interpretations can occur when you have experienced some event and you falsely attribute an unrelated reason as the cause. From then on, that becomes an unwritten rule for you moving forward—though it is inaccurate. For example, maybe you finally made it back to the gym but misplaced your membership card and the front desk person was having a bad day and was nasty to you. Perhaps you incorrectly interpreted their rudeness as them judging you or judging how you looked, so now you no longer go to the gym. Another example, maybe you start to share your vision and health goals with others close to you. As you share with excitement, you see minimum reaction or perhaps receive a few negative comments. Maybe your inspiration causes them to feel like they are not where they want to be. Instead of recognizing that, you misinterpret it as them thinking that your goals are not possible or worthwhile, so you give up before even trying.

Limiting Beliefs: Assumptions from the Past

Beliefs are created when we mistakenly assume that because a similar event happened in the past, it will have the same outcome in the present or future. This is what I mean about a limiting belief that is an assumption from the past. For example, you tried an exercise in the past like spinning and you got hurt, so you decide you will no longer exercise with a bicycle because you will get hurt. This is not an accurate conclusion and one that limits you from reaching better health. Learning from your past is an incredibly valuable skill, but making a life completely limited by your past is not.

Limiting Beliefs: Deep-Seated Beliefs

Deep-seated beliefs, at their core, are ones that tell us that we are not good enough. Perhaps not good enough to deserve good health or a good life. Just before we are about to embark on something big, we all have had a little voice inside that heckles us, saying, "Who do you think you are to go for that?" We all have deep-seated limiting beliefs, and these have often separated us from our highest goals. They tend to show up right when we are about to step towards our greatness, when we are reaching for what is possible. Tell that little doubting voice that you got this and make sure you take that first step. The key to squashing this type of belief is consistent positive self-talk, recognition that you have been successful in other endeavors, and taking action.

What is possible in your life is a direct reflection of the beliefs you have about your life.

Declaring New Possibilities

Once you start recognizing limiting beliefs by increasing your awareness of them, you can begin the journey of replacing them with empowering beliefs. Declaring a new possibility, a new empowering belief, sets your belief system and life in motion for optimal healthy living. An example could be:

My old limiting belief was that all exercise was _____ [examples: hard, painful, boring, time-consuming].

My new possibility, that I am inventing for myself and my life, is the possibility of exercise being _____ [examples: energizing, exciting, rewarding].

Synergy Action Steps

The aim of the following steps is for you to bring your limiting beliefs to the surface and then eradicate them. Most of the time they were formed unconsciously at a young, less mature stage of your life and you were blind to their formation. Expect to have to repeat the process given in the following steps for eradicating limiting beliefs several times because you more than likely have several dominant limiting beliefs that are robbing you from achieving your ultimate health. Here are the steps for eradicating your limiting beliefs:

1. When you are moving forward in your health, ask yourself, "What are my beliefs about my health?"

2. To determine if it is a limiting belief ask, "Is this particular belief expanding my capacity or limiting my health potential?"

3. If it is a limiting belief, identify which category of the four limiting beliefs it falls into: generalities, false interpretations, assumptions from the past, or deep-seated beliefs.

4. Create a shift in your belief pattern. Ask yourself some empowering questions:

   a. For generalities: does this belief happen all the time and every single time, or am I making a global generalization?

   b. For false interpretations: what are some OTHER empowering meanings I can gain from that past experience?

   c. For assumptions from the past: does my past always equal my future? What other things have happened to me in the past where I was able to successfully shift my approach and get a different result?

   d. For deep-seated beliefs: what is something I can tell that little voice of doubt that will cause it to shut its mouth? What are some affirmations I can say out loud and to myself that encourage me and that are louder than that little doubting voice? The key is to understand that these doubting voices inevitably are going to show up and to remind yourself of all the elements within the Synergy Success Cycle.

5. Take immediate action and produce results that shatter the limiting belief.

6. Recognize when you achieve success beyond your initial limiting belief. At that moment, declare a new empowering belief as described above.

7. Reward yourself with something positive to highlight your progress.

8. Remind yourself of this success the next time you see that limiting belief creep in.

CHAPTER 9

Q1 POWER—RULES

*The rules you create for your life, either consciously
or unconsciously, shape the quality of your life.
Change your rules and you change your life.*

—Dr. Eric Janowitz

Rules, according to the *Oxford Dictionary*, are defined as "one of a set of explicit or understood regulations or principles governing conduct within a particular activity or sphere." Because they are a set of principles governing a particular thing, there exists the possibility for our values, viewpoints, talents, beliefs, and limiting beliefs to shape our rules. This is actually a very good thing because as you progress and repeat the Synergy Success Cycle throughout your life, you can see that your rules can serve to create an increased quality of life.

Specifically, let's examine some of your rules relating to health. Please complete the following sentences with just a few words to gain more clarity on the rules you have created in your life regarding each of the following important aspects of health. Don't overthink it, just write or say whatever comes first to your mind:

- *Health is _____.*
- *Exercise is _____.*
- *Healing comes from _____.*
- *My ideal weight is _____.*
- *With healthy living, I can live to _____.*

When you complete the sentences above, try taking a look at your responses as if someone else wrote them. What would you say that person believes about these areas? If someone says exercise is hard, what would you think that person's level of engagement would be in that activity? Starting to uncover your rules for what "rings the bell" for success or what things mean, helps you further clarify what you presently believe, not only about the area, but also your values, viewpoint, beliefs, and limiting beliefs.

The "Acting As If" Rule

Other rules can often dictate how to feel emotionally, which can send us into a positive or negative state as we are striving to increase our power (Q1). They could look something like:

- *In order to feel _____, I must _____.*

This means that for you to, say, reward yourself with a positive feeling of happiness, you must first do something and will only allow yourself to feel happiness depending on the success of doing that identified thing (i.e., the rule you created). The problem with this kind of rule is that it sets you up for failure. It's all-or-nothing with no nuances or gray areas. It emphasizes the destination when, in fact, in order to engage with an activity consistently, you must appreciate its journey, the actual doing of it.

What if we looked at the emotions created from our rules differently? How about this equation:

1. *If I was to successfully perform/complete* _____ [activity],
2. *I would **feel** _____* [new empowering emotion].
3. *If I were to feel a sense of* _____ [new empowering emotion] *on a consistent basis,*
4. *that would create a state of **being** _____.*

Think about this: our sense of "being" comes from experiencing a consistent emotional pattern. When we look from the lens of the power quadrant, we desire to become more powerful in directing and influencing our lives. **It is important to recognize and clearly identify the person you are becoming as you move through the Synergy Success Cycle.** As you move into it positively, your sense of being can include such examples as whole, complete, peaceful, refreshed, energized, or healthy.

5. *I will, therefore, approach* _____ [future activity] *with a state of being _____.*

This means approaching the future activity with the mindset of a state of being that is more powerful than the default limiting emotional pattern you have used prior in your life. This is an example of "acting as if" the goal was already accomplished and entering the activity already with the emotional reward of strength and certainty. For example, imagine if you were to enter the game of life with the mindset that you had already won.

Here is an example: *In order to feel happy, I must exercise 30 minutes every day.* Great statement, and you probably will feel happy if you do that. But what if you miss a day? No happiness rewards? How long will that habit last and keep you motivated for the reward if you have a few missed days in a row?

I recommend changing your approach to this: *If I were to successfully complete 30 minutes of exercise every day, I would feel happy. If I were to feel a sense of happiness on a consistent basis, that would create a state of being peaceful and confident.*

Now how much better would your approach and your satisfaction to exercising 30 minutes per day become if you were beginning the exercise and executing it while already being in a state of peacefulness and confidence? The point is that while most people's "rule" is to *wait* for the *completion* of the activity to give them the emotional reward, you don't have to do this. By abiding by the "acting as if" rule, you already allow yourself to experience the emotional award such that you encourage yourself to engage more consistently (consistency being a key to health) with the activity (i.e., process, Q4).

I should add that in reality, each of us always wins in life because in every experience there is a lesson to be learned and an opportunity for growth whether we seemed to "win" or "lose." I recommend making this one of your life rules too!

For most people, initiating the health activity is the hard part, so if we can start healthy lifestyle activities with the positive emotional state already engaged in our nervous system, we are more likely to create the momentum to provide the health benefits of the activity.

Synergy Action Steps

1. Did you think about or write down some of your health rules? If you haven't, please do so.
2. What did you learn about yourself when examining your rules for healthy living?
3. What new rules can you create in your life that can take your health to the next level? Make sure to consider some new "acting as if" rules here as well.

CHAPTER 10

Q1 POWER—REFLECTION, VICTORIES, AND CELEBRATIONS

The more you praise and celebrate your life, the more there is in life to celebrate.

—Oprah Winfrey

As an achiever, I have long considered myself someone who prides himself on getting things done in a powerful way and at an extraordinary rate. I often find myself guilty of being laser-focused on a project, only to complete it and allow myself a cursory pat on the back before I quickly move on to the next task at hand. Are you guilty of that? Most achievers are.

I have learned over the years, however, how critical reflection is to the human mind, body, and spirit. When you are always focusing on and only handling the situations of day-to-day life, you are reacting to the current demands. You are not reflecting on the big picture of what's happening, so you can fail to learn the lessons in life's experiences. Reflection requires time allocation and practice. People reflect in different ways—some write, others quietly reflect, and others verbalize.

Who you ultimately become is related to the quality of the reflection you give yourself. We are not human *doings*, but rather human *beings*. Becoming the person you want to be involves having experiences and taking the time to reflect on what those experiences mean in your life. Reflection allows you to see how your experiences align with or go against your values. These experiences not only shape your beliefs, life, and the world around you, but equally important, if not more so, they shape the beliefs you have about yourself.

On a scale of one to ten, how satisfied are you with your current level of health? What specifically did you think about to help you come up with that number? Some people look at their body weight. Others their activity level. Still others consider the pain they are experiencing. Others could have poor posture. Others may be dealing with a chronic health condition like diabetes or cancer.

Let's go back in time. Can you reflect on a time when you were at your ideal body weight? How were you living at that time? What were the consistent things you were doing at that time (i.e., your habits)? What activities did you engage in that brought you happiness and joy? What was life like prior to managing a chronic illness? What things did you enjoy then and with whom?

How did you "celebrate" life back then? How do you celebrate life now? What are your recent health accomplishments? Have you stopped rewarding yourself for your recent health accomplishments? Are you in need of setting some new health goals (ones we will cover in purpose, Q2)?

Reflection: Near-Event and Long-Term

Reflection is like that syrupy chocolate topping that molds and hardens when it makes contact with cold ice cream. The molding of the chocolate shell occurs best when the ice cream is at its coldest. Reflection should also occur in close proximity to the time of the event when the event is fresh in your mind. This is why something as simple as a gratitude journal used each night to denote three things you are grateful for is so useful. When you reflect later that evening or the next day, you can still elicit the emotions you felt. You can use those emotions as a guide to help you gain a better understanding of the lessons from that experience. You should insert a quick "near-event" reflection period in your life. This is especially important with your health because this is an area where you can be most hard on yourself. Instead of reminding yourself of what you were not able to enjoy with your lowered health state, seek ways to see what you were able to do and experience gratitude. Near-event reflection is important because it connects you better to the emotional states you experienced, which can serve as a guidepost for you.

Long-term reflection is also important because it helps you to see who you have become over time. You don't become overweight, fatigued, or depressed overnight. You also don't become healthy, vibrant, and happy overnight either. Long-term reflection is best done on a quarterly basis and an annual basis. Just as a healthy functioning business needs to take inventory on what is working and not working on a regular basis, a healthy functioning body and mind need the same discipline. Long-term reflection helps you see why you may have had an emotional response to a particular situation and who you are becoming, and it gives you significantly greater clarity on what's important to you and why.

There is an abundant amount of journaling books in the marketplace to help you with reflecting, celebrating, and planning. The problem is that most planners do not cover all the components that the Synergy Life system utilizes. We are developing our unique **Synergy Life Plan Journal** to ensure you cover all the bases for capturing all 4 Ps.

Please express your interest in the Synergy Life Plan Journal by contacting us through our website www.TheSynergyLife.com.

Celebrate!

Besides reflecting, we need to celebrate. A celebration is a perfect way to make an exclamation point on accomplishment. I notice that many adults do not know how to celebrate anymore. Look and see how many adults like to celebrate birthdays! You don't often see adults gathered around for a pool party with their friends to celebrate their birthdays. They are not sharing a pizza, singing "Happy Birthday" with a cake flooded with enough candles to light up the street, their favorite music in the background, and everybody leaving with a goodie bag of powdery sugar sweets. When was the last time you truly celebrated something in your life? I mean, really celebrated?

If you don't create an *intention* to celebrate in your life, it will not happen. What are some things that you're working on right now that once you complete them, they are worth celebrating? Can what you are working on be broken down into smaller milestones where each of them has some little celebration?

Small celebrations for everyday victories do not need to be huge. The key is finding a way to put an exclamation point, metaphorically speaking, on different events in your life. You will not remember all the moments in your life, but you will remember significant ones. The more you make those moments "celebration points," the deeper those memories will be instilled in your nervous system, your physiology, your heart, and your spirit.

When we think of the past, we want to feel positive emotions because of the progress we have made. That is what celebrations of our victories create—a greater emphasis on the positive events that moved us forward in life. If you are targeting your ideal weight, can you break it into quarters, so every time you reach one quarter closer to your goal, you celebrate? If you want to lose 40 pounds, create some celebration for every ten pounds you lose that gets you closer to your 40 pound goal. What can some celebrations look like? How about a celebratory healthy lunch with friends? How about a reward of a new book, kitchen device, or outfit? When you reach your big goal, make the celebration more special. I found that a change in scenery often is a good pattern interruption to make a celebration memorable. Perhaps a quick weekend getaway at a nearby resort? A visit to a friend or family member that you have been wanting to connect with?

In reality, though, most people reflect on their past and only see the losses that have stacked up over time. This kind of reflection results in us beating ourselves up, and it creates limiting beliefs and interferes with our ability to fully express our best life ever. This type of reflection dims the light of possibility and slows down the Synergy Success Cycle.

So, what we do in response to stacked adverse events? When I did my professional coach training, they first wanted us to make a clear distinction between coaching an individual versus providing therapy. Coaching is about recognizing our past, understanding the choices that we can currently make, and creating an empowering future. Coaching is more about working in the present and working on the future.

Therapy, on the other hand, is more about healing the past. We all have had significant events in our history, and some of them have severely negatively impacted who we are. Some have resulted in deep scars and painful wounds. For those people who have been held hostage by negative, destructive thoughts and behavior patterns, seeing a professional therapist is a critical investment in their health and life. Every day that you are stuck in the past you are losing your today. I encourage you to get help from a professional if you are past-driven and can't get unstuck on your own.

A Funeral for Past Failures

If you have successfully made it through a negative event and reflected on the lessons learned, then having a "funeral" for that event can be a good strategy to close that chapter and move on. For example, I made a terrible real estate investment decision in my early, immature years of investing. I managed to buy one of the worst pieces of real estate investment vehicles. I purchased a property that managed to lose 90% of its value in a matter of two years! I prided myself on my ability to make good decisions, so making this poor decision involving bad real estate timing shook me at the core. It rattled my self-confidence in my ability to make good decisions not only in real estate but spilled over into other areas of my life. Many of the people who also fell victim to similar poor real estate investments ended up with devastating effects in their lives. I read of people getting divorced, having heart attacks, and some even taking their own life.

What did I do to rid myself of these negative emotional patterns that resulted from this lousy investment? I created a funeral, metaphorically speaking, for this experience. What I mean by that is that I had to go through the process of burying the bad decision, grieving the loss of not only the money, but more importantly, the deeper feeling that I'd made a poor decision. I had to bury the guilt it caused for not only myself but for my family. I screamed and cried to release the negative emotions. After I let the negative emotions free from my body, I was able to detach myself from that situation and take a step back to create *new* empowering *meanings* from this event.

By losing so much money but working through this painful long nightmare with my wife, I reflected and, therefore, allowed myself to receive tremendous gifts from this event. I created a powerful belief that I can get through anything. I also created the powerful belief that my wife and I are a fantastic team, and life or situations will not get us down. I also became less attached to money because I learned how easy it can come and how fast one decision can take it away. In talking with other successful people and sharing my story, I discovered that most millionaires have lost significant fortunes in their lives with certain investments. I learned, in fact, many of them that I have met have actually gone through bankruptcy.

When you look back at your beliefs, think of the state you were in and the feelings you were experiencing when you formed them. Where do you need to have a funeral for something in your past? Where is there an opportunity to release the negative emotions around that event and allow yourself to create a new, fresh, exciting perspective and empowering beliefs?

Your sense of personal power is a combination of your strengths, values, viewpoint, beliefs, limiting beliefs, rules, victories, and celebrations. Reflection is a potent tool to clarify these concepts along your life's journey. Your sense of personal power creates your self-identity and establishes your level of confidence in each area of your life. Your current level of personal power will serve as the foundation of establishing your purpose, quadrant 2, which we turn to in the next chapter. Again, your level of health purpose will rise and fall based on the level of your self-confidence and your sense of power (Q1) in regards to your health. Power and purpose, both of which are part of your inner work, are what is necessary to set the stage for the external manifestation of unlocking and experiencing your best health.

Synergy Action Steps

1. When was the last time you truly celebrated your health accomplishments?
2. What are some health celebrations you can add to your life? With whom? Can they be broken down into some mini-celebrations along the way?
3. What failure might you need to have a funeral for, so you can move on with your health and life?

QUADRANT 2— PURPOSE

Purpose is the fuel for the fire of your life. Most people know that purpose is important in creating an outstanding life, but they often lack the clarity or tools to tap into it. In these next chapters, you'll be looking at your purpose in these terms:

- Chapter 11: your purpose in terms of your "compelling" why
- Chapter 12: your purpose in terms of your ultimate vision
- Chapter 13: your purpose in terms of your inspiring goals

When you become clear on your purpose, vision, and goals, then the magic happens. Like a magnet, you start to recognize and attract people (Q3) that are consistent with your dominant thought patterns. Since purpose, vision, and goals are highly charged emotionally, they serve as the best magnet to attract people (Q3) who are in alignment with you, which in turn propels you farther along the Synergy Success Cycle. As a result, you establish an incredibly strong framework, so that your health is optimized as well. When you put synergy to work in your favor, you create a win-win feedback loop for your health, yourself, and your life overall.

CHAPTER 11

Q2 PURPOSE— COMPELLING "WHY"

This is the true joy in life, being used for a purpose recognized by yourself as a mighty one. Being a force of nature instead of a feverish, selfish little clod of ailments and grievances, complaining that the world will not devote itself to making you happy. I am of the opinion that my life belongs to the whole community and as long as I live, it is my privilege to do for it what I can. I want to be thoroughly used up when I die, for the harder I work, the more I live. I rejoice in life for its own sake. Life is no brief candle to me. It is a sort of splendid torch which I have got hold of for the moment and I want to make it burn as brightly as possible before handing it on to future generations.

—George Bernard Shaw

The definition of "purpose" is the reason for which something is done or created, or for which something exists. In relationship to you, it is your compelling "why," your ultimate vision, and your inspiring goals. To achieve anything of greatness, I believe you have to have a clear sense of the compelling reason why you're doing it. Your why is your fuel to get you through the hard times as well as serving as your internal compass to give you direction.

Regaining health is much harder after it is lost than simply maintaining it. To regain our health once again, we must deeply connect to our purpose on why we want to be healthy. The harder the health goal and health challenges to overcome, the greater your purpose has to become.

Small Health Goals = A Small Purpose Required

Large Health Goals = A Clear, Emotionally Compelling Purpose Required

While I've already shared how and why I became a chiropractor, there are some parts of that story I want to revisit to highlight the significance of having a purpose and a compelling why.

When I was going through chiropractic college, I knew that I wanted to have a large family practice. Because I'd dealt with my own back struggles, I'd created a negative belief that my physical body was weak. Ironically, my personal back issues were the catalyst for creating my big why. I wanted to help other people by inspiring them to see themselves as greater than their current reality and by providing them a solution to strengthen their perceived weaknesses.

A chiropractor's role is to release nerve interference for the purpose of allowing the body to fully express its maximum health potential. Chiropractic appreciates that the body is designed to heal and thrive. Your body is designed to fully express its health and greatness. I globally designed my approach to patient care to help patients achieve greatness in all areas of their lives. I not only wanted to reduce the nerve interference in their spine, but also the interference they had in areas that limited their sense of Q1 power. I wanted to give them an adjustment of hope in their life and help them at least recognize the potential within themselves. I wanted them to use their full potential to impact the people in their lives positively. In fact, it was the chiropractic philosophy of removing interference to allow greatness to naturally express itself that was the foundation for this entire book.

My goal and purpose were to help people eliminate the barriers within their physical and mental health to allow them to fully express the life they were meant to have. Because I knew at a young age that I wanted to be a chiropractor, I was able to enter chiropractic school with an incredibly compelling why.

As already mentioned, in my senior year, I went to high school in the morning and after lunch would intern in my chiropractor's office. I would help with simple administrative tasks such as filing, but as the team saw my continued interest, they added more opportunities for me to learn and grow. I created my first mini-book in high school, a ten-page booklet explaining the power of the nervous system and chiropractic. This booklet was given to all new patients who entered the practice. I also helped the clinical assistants by putting patients on the physical therapy machines.

When I shadowed Dr. Elliott, I would hear story after story of patients telling me how chiropractic changed their lives. I remember hearing a firefighter share that he fell out of a three-story building, and if it weren't for chiropractic, he would not be able to walk. I remember parents telling me about their children continually getting sick until they found the chiropractic approach. I remember seeing pictures, posters, and sports memorabilia of famous actors and athletes thanking Dr. Elliott for the care he provided. I remember too just how much Dr. Elliott's patients cared for him as their healer and how much he genuinely and positively cared for them. Every time I saw him make a positive, heartfelt connection with his patients, it reminded me of the time that I received this love from him as a nine-year-old receiving treatments. Every encounter with the hundreds of patients I witnessed reinforced the reason why I decided to do this type of work. It became a mission for me to be the best chiropractor possible.

After graduating chiropractic college, as already mentioned, I found the busiest chiropractic office in Orlando that shared both my same strong belief in the chiropractic principles of healing and in life. About six months into that practice, I discovered another circle of chiropractors (people, Q3) who had an even bigger vision and compelling why (Q2). One chiropractor in particular, Dr. Dan Yachter, was serving twice the number of patients that my busy practice was serving. I didn't think it was possible to see that many patients and deliver high-quality care. My limiting beliefs system (Q1) was eradicated after observing the processes and quality of care and patient satisfaction of Dr. Dan's practice.

I decided to work for Dr. Dan's practice on Thursdays, my day off, without pay, simply to be around a practice that had this significant compelling why and learn how they did it. Developing my why was worth more to me than any financial gain I would've received working for that practice or for the free time I sacrificed as a result of being exposed to that environment.

When you reflect on your life's history and what is important to you, how do you currently see your purpose tied into becoming even more healthy and achieving your best health? When you are confronting a healthy activity that you don't necessarily want to do but know is important, what greater purpose are you connecting it with? We are all providers at some level to others in our lives. It could be children, aging parents, co-workers, or the people we serve. Rather than just unconsciously performing helpful activities for these people, begin the process of increasing your awareness on why you need to be healthy not only for yourself, but also for those around you.

The Rule of 5/7

Most people work five days a week. Most people hate Mondays and love Fridays. They live by a limiting belief (Q1) that work is work and play is play. Working is often associated with taking away from what they want to do, and it is considered something they have to do. When you have to do something, it feels like work, not passion. No one is passionate about having to do something that is forced upon them.

The rule of 5/7 simply means that if you don't like what you do for a living (5 days in your week), then 5/7 of your life sucks. That means the majority of your life sucks. The 5/7 rule says that if you're doing what you don't like to do for a majority of the time, then it is literally sucking the life out of you. In truth, if 5/7 of your life sucks, then there's a good chance that you won't be as successful and will probably become negative, which puts a lot of stress on you, which in turn can manifest itself as poor health … so the other 2/7 of your life will also suck. This means 7 out of 7 of your life sucks!

I apologize if my choice of words offends you, but I am using this language to make my point clear. Rather than being disturbed by my intentional use of the word "suck," you should be more disturbed if you are not living a life you deserve to live. A life of joy, happiness, fulfillment, purpose, inspiration, goals, passion, energy, and health. Now that doesn't suck!

To the degree that you can find a compelling why in the areas of your life, specifically your health, is the degree that you will fully connect with the right people and engage the actions necessary to achieve results of significance. This is the Synergy Success Cycle in action!

What is your compelling why to be healthy? Is your compelling why focused on yourself, or is it for others? Another way of asking this question: does your purpose go beyond the purpose tipping point from self to others? You see, I would make a lot of poor food choices if I was just satisfying my own desire to eat food that gives me pleasure. I really don't like exercise. I personally am not very motivated to work out on a consistent basis. If left to my own devices, I would let my email and other office "demands" consume my weekdays, which would leave me little time to exercise.

However, due to my compelling why, which involves others, I don't give in to these less-than-optimal health choices. I want to be the best chiropractor possible. I have a standard that I want my level of expertise, energy, and engagement to be just as high for my last patient of the day as compared to the first patient I see in the morning. To do this, I know that I need strength, endurance, and energy. I know that exercise, a positive mental attitude, and healthy food are critical. I would not work out or eat a mostly plant-based diet for myself, but I will for my patients and I will to be a better leader of my team. I will eat anything convenient and fast (which is likely unhealthy) for myself, but I will eat better foods to have better energy in order to care for others. **My health area expands and improves to the degree that my reason for doing it expands and improves.**

I was a stutterer when I was a child. I remember being in middle school where the teacher would have people read sentences one by one, going up and down the rows. I remember secretly counting up and down the rows to determine the exact sentence that I had to read. I knew the information and answers, but I was afraid that I would not be able to get the words out of my mouth and how it would make me look. I remember fear overcoming my whole body and my palms sweating when I saw that the particular sentence I was to read began with the letter M. Ms were difficult for me to say. Instead, I played dumb and pretended that

I was not paying attention and was lost in what the teacher was teaching simply to avoid having to read those sentences out loud. Back then, I chose to play small because I was worried about how I would look to my peers. I was focused on myself. My purpose was focused on myself and just making it through the class without attention.

After exposing myself to the power of chiropractic and the effect it had on so many lives, I increased my belief in my potential and my purpose. My life shifted and literally transformed. When my purpose became greater than myself, I got out of my own way. Now I am a regular public speaker. As opposed to avoiding and retreating from situations like speaking, I actively seek them out. I know that the message of increased life and health potential is far more valuable than the fears that I have around looking good.

When you communicate to yourself and others from a sense of power and purpose (Q1 and Q2), you simply get out of your own way. When you communicate to yourself and others with a sense of power and purpose, the message becomes greater than the messenger. You then are just a vessel for your mission and purpose. This, my friend, creates a life that includes hard work because your mission is huge, but it also includes a life of fulfillment.

The Gift in Your Struggle

People oftentimes struggle with discovering their compelling why. This esoteric thing is something that people deeply desire but have a lot of uncertainty around discovering. Just like in getting clarity on your values, I believe discovering your why begins by analyzing the high points and low points of your life. It is in the peaks and valleys where you really learn about yourself and what is important to you.

We have all been beaten up and knocked down in life. We have had actions happen around us that conflict with our values. We have all made poor health choices that caught up to us. Don't waste a good struggle in your life. When something beats you down emotionally, look at it as if you were an outside observer. As that observer, ask yourself what it was about that experience that really affected you emotionally. What does this mean? Where is the gift in this? What does this tell you about yourself? Can you discover a greater meaning, that the event revealed, that gives you a sense of increased responsibility, a sense of purpose to make sure that thing will not happen again? Besides simply feeling your emotions and letting them run your life, use your emotions to discover more about what makes you tick and what gets you excited. How can you use that excitement to help yourself and those around you?

The Gift in Your Victories

You should not only look at the lows in your life but also the highs. Anytime you are in a peak state emotionally, open your eyes, heart, intellect, and intuition. We all have victories, but a few select ones really charge and inspire us. In those experiences, you should definitely reflect on what aspect of that experience you became deeply connected to. Ask yourself, "In this victory, what about it did I deeply connect to? How does this event shed light on how I can effectively make my mark on this world?"

In regards to your health, there are certainly high and low points. In looking at both sides of the equation be sure to see your greater why. Be sure to start linking your why to your desire to be healthy. When you are about to start a tough health activity or make a good health choice, remind yourself, "I am doing this because …"

Synergy Action Steps

1. What is your compelling why to be healthy?
2. Is your compelling why focused on yourself, or is it focused on others?
3. In looking at your highs and lows in health and life, what do you learn about your purpose for achieving your best health?
4. What can you do to remind yourself on a consistent basis of your why to be healthy?

CHAPTER 12

Q2 PURPOSE— ULTIMATE VISION

Where there is no vision, the people perish.

—Proverbs 29:18

Once you start to get a sense of your compelling why, then your vision for what you want starts to crystallize, and the creative process begins. You need a vision for what you want. You need to create in your mind a firm picture of your desired outcomes. You can want to have good health and have a reason for it, but if you don't know what that will look like, then it will lack sustainability.

When you look at your health today, how does it compare to your ideal vision? Most would say that it does not. The problem is that most people are very clear about what they *don't* want for their health, but very few people have the clarity of knowing their ideal vision for their health.

Instead of first visualizing what you want for your health, let's first examine how you visualize. When you visualize how you want something to be, how do you process it? What is your preferred style for visioning? Ideally, you should have a grasp on the best way you can create a clear picture of what you want. This will make it significantly easier to visualize your desired outcomes.

Because we are talking about vision creating, most initially think that we must use a visual mode, the mode that visual learners prefer. Visual learners learn best by seeing things either in the real world or in their minds. They have a preference for using imagery, pictures, or video to understand or create content—i.e., visual visioning.

Visual learners might visualize best by creating vision boards. A vision board consists of a series of images from magazines, newspapers, the internet, etc., that depict your ideal vision for an area of your life. For finances, it may be a future bank statement showing the future balance you aim for or pictures of cars or homes that you desire. Visual learners would then post their vision board where they will see it often, so their conscious and unconscious have lots of exposure to it. Visual people also respond well to posting inspiring quotes, phrases, or icons around them. I have put quotes on the bottom of my computer screen, in my bathroom mirror, and on the rearview mirror of my car. Some even decorate their laptop with images of their desired outcome. My screensaver in college said, "Make it happen" or "Whatever it takes," to serve as a constant visual reminder of the persistence I wanted in order to reach my bigger goals.

Your brain "sees" what you see when your eyes collect physical images of your environment, but it also "sees" by envisioning images that it constructs. Your body can literally feel the same sensations from input in both modes, input that is seen in the outside world and input constructed inside the mind. I remember first being exposed to this concept by the sports psychology book *The Inner Game of Tennis*. In this classic book, it explains that people who were not able to play tennis due to injury took time away from the court and instead visualized themselves playing the game of tennis in their mind. They would visualize themselves tossing the ball up perfectly for a serve, bringing their arm back, and crushing the ball in the sweet spot of the racket. They could literally feel in their mind the sensation of that perfect hit, the sound it made, the sensation the racket created in their wrist from the impact, and the ease and speed at which the ball left the strings. They could then visualize the ball landing perfectly with the precise spin they desired. Research found that athletes that actively visualized themselves participating in their sport, even when sidelined, often retained their skill set and sharpness once they returned to action, as compared to those who left the court and did not visualize. Again, the brain is powerful, so let's apply that power to our advantage. I encourage you to envision yourself putting into action the processes (Q4) to achieve your best health and visualizing yourself as you look and feel when in great health.

Daydreaming is often frowned upon in school, but it can serve as another helpful source of visioning. Personally, I do some of my best visioning while taking a shower. This is one of my quiet times away from the demands of the practice and my family. During this time, I allow myself to get lost in my thoughts, which allows me to problem solve and usually ends with me creating a vision in my head about a desired outcome. I often won't stop my shower until I have a clear view of the solution and feel a sense of accomplishment because I see the problem already handled. Some showers can be quite long!

Others visualize with their ears and mouth. Learning from your ears is the aural mode. Sounds brought to the ears are processed in a part of the brain called Wernicke's area. This is different from the part of the brain that processes a person's own spoken words, which is Broca's area. This distinction is important to point out because although they are both auditory in mode, processing from hearing someone else speak versus processing from speaking yourself happens in different parts of the brain. I am a big fan of audiobooks. I listen to books (aural learning) more often than I physically read books (visual). I love hearing authors read their own books because you can often hear not only the words but the emotional state they were in when they wrote the words. When listening (as opposed to reading), I am better adept at feeling the emotion behind the words, so I gain a deeper meaning of the message.

That is quite different than using speaking or verbal communication as a means of processing. You may be the type of person who gains clarity of vision by talking about your dreams and visions to others. In this case, creating intentional times to meet with others who are supportive of your ideas and offer positive constructive criticism are essential to formulating your ideas. My wife learns by reading books and then tells me how she wants to integrate the ideas in her life. This offers her a way to create clarity of vision.

Another way I gain clarity is creating talks with PowerPoint and visually designing the slides as well as sequencing the slides in a format that flows for me to express my ideas. I run through the slides and speak in my mind the concepts I want to convey (a form of internal verbal communication similar to the tennis player visually playing the game in their mind). Then I teach the concepts with verbal communication where I can see the body language of the audience and listen to and handle their questions. I typically end a presentation by asking the audience to do a 15-second share of what "hit them between the eyes." This verbal, visual, and aural dance of communication allows me to "visualize" the concepts I am creating.

You may be more of a kinesthetic learner. These learners learn by physically doing. Some of you will solidify your vision by "putting the cook in the kitchen." Physically doing the activity you see yourself wanting to do as part of your ultimate vision not only creates momentum in starting action towards your desire, it also allows you to physically feel the activity. This feeling can serve as a valuable feedback system to see if the activity resonates with your vision and at the same time allows you to finetune it.

While my first chiropractic office was being built, I lived in a small one-bedroom apartment. I put a large blueprint of my future office, which showed all the rooms mapped out, above my small dining room table. At 27 years old, I remember regularly eating dinner by myself and staring at the blueprints. I visualized myself going into each of the treatment rooms, one after the other, and I would see myself adjusting patients. I felt my hands pressing gently across their backs and palpating their spines. I remember placing the proper hand contact on their back in the area that needed correction. I recall breathing with the patient and gently applying the corrective force to release the nerve pressure. I felt the connection I had with each patient in each room as I left them in a better state to heal than when they walked in. I would see ten to twenty patients in my mind each time I ate dinner. It felt just as real as doing it physically. While this was going on, I visualized the things my team would communicate with patients, the music that was playing, the positive energy, and even the colors of the office.

Later on, when my practice was ready to get going, I simply matched the real office to the office that I'd envisioned in my mind from those hundreds of visualization sessions over dinner. As Napoleon Hill stated so eloquently, "Whatever the mind can conceive and believe, it can achieve."

Looking at this from the lens of the Synergy Success Cycle, the mind "believing" is the power quadrant (Q2). If you do not believe you have the talent or capacity to achieve a health vision of what you want, then there is a disconnect and it will not happen. Said another way, the level of your belief in achieving your optimal health (or something else) will dictate the level of your ultimate vision. Your capacity to believe in yourself and your overall power determines—either for the best or worst—the reach of your vision of what is possible. Again, that is why the Synergy Success Cycle starts with YOU, identifying your strengths, values, viewpoint, beliefs, and rules (Q1). Understanding yourself sets the foundation for creating the vision for how and why you want to impact this world (Q2). Understanding YOU allows you to visualize what kind of health you want to achieve.

State-Dependent Theory

Another important psychological principle is called state-dependent theory. State-dependent theory explains that memory retrieval is most effective and efficient when an individual is in the same state of consciousness as they were when the memory was formed. This means that we need to be aware of our physiology when we are creating our vision. Physiology is the study of how the body normally moves and functions. You want to be very intentional *when* you visualize. Getting yourself in a positive, energized, and upbeat mood, or state, really helps to lock in your vision. Think of your senses when engaging in the creation of your vision for your optimal health. Getting your body in motion, such as running or cycling, while creating the vision in your mind is powerful to many people. Listening to upbeat music and dancing around is another way to fill the body, mind, and spirit, and integrate them while forming your vision. You can also think of yourself as a calm warrior who meditates and sits with strong posture while breathing intentionally with eyes closed and chest upright as they see or hear themselves confidently pursuing their vision. Others incorporate the use of smell such as rubbing essential oils on their wrists and breathing in deeply as they create their ideal vision.

Psychologists have proven that when people are learning in a peak state, their learning goes deeper into their nervous system.

Psychologists have also proven that when people get back into these peak states, they are able to go back to the place in their mind where their ultimate vision was created. That is the state-dependent theory, and you should be conscious of using it and manipulating your environment and your own physiology in creating your vision for your optimal health.

Begin the process today of reshaping and retooling your ultimate vision for your health using your ideal modes of visualizing and learning. Then find strategies to put in your calendar and in your environment to help you increase your exposure to this vision of optimal health on a repetitive and consistent basis. This internal work will serve as the foundation to the second half of the Synergy Success Cycle, the outer expression, where you attract the right people (Q3) into your life as well as enact the best processes (Q4) to obtain your desired results.

Synergy Action Steps

1. Which modes of learning do you best connect with? Which do you use most often with success? Again, it is important to know the "code behind the code." It is by understanding how you learn that will increase your capacity to learn more efficiently, effectively, and impactfully.

2. What is your ideal vision of your health? Consider looking at your health as seasons. In two seasons, or six months, what is your vision of ultimate health? Does it consist of an ideal weight, body fat percentage, posture, or strength capacity? Is it fitting into a certain type or size of clothing? How well does your body move? Do your joints move freely and without pain? Are you walking with a certain confidence in your step? Are you flexible and limber? Are you standing tall with a powerful posture? What foods are on your plate? How are you nourishing yourself? Describe your sleep.

3. How about your energy when you are at your optimal health? What does your ideal energy look like? How does it feel? How will you know you have achieved your ideal energy? What is your barometer? With this ideal energy, physical strength, and vitality, what activities do you see yourself doing and enjoying even more of?

4. How does your ideal health state translate into your relationship with your spouse (including intimacy), children, friends, coworkers, and other key people in your life?

Q2 PURPOSE— INSPIRING GOALS

The tragedy of life doesn't lie in not reaching your goal. The tragedy lies in having no goal to reach. It isn't a calamity to die with dreams unfulfilled, but it is a calamity not to dream ... It is not a disgrace not to reach the stars, but it is a disgrace to have no stars to reach for. Not failure, but low aim is sin.

—Benjamin Mays, American minister
and mentor to Dr. Martin Luther King Jr.

We have already discussed the need to have a compelling why and the importance of knowing the reasons behind what you want. This is the fuel for achieving your optimum health as well as realizing any dream you have in life.

Your ultimate vision is the creative process of finding your best way to see the desired outcome. Your inspiring goals then serve as the small and large guideposts along the journey of achieving your ultimate vision. There exists some new compelling scientific research on goalsetting and the specifics on best achieving goals.

Gail Matthews led a groundbreaking research study around goal setting.[16] The study's participants were broken into five groups. The first group was simply asked to *think about* the goals that they wanted to accomplish in a month and to rate each goal according to the following criteria:

- Difficulty, importance, the extent to which they had the skills and resources to accomplish the goals (i.e., their power, Q1),
- Their commitment and motivation (i.e., their compelling why, Q2), and
- Whether they had pursued the goal before and if so, their prior success (i.e., this is the completion of one revolution of the Synergy Success Cycle that reinforces a person's power (Q1) and, thus, starts a new Synergy Success Cycle).

The second group was asked to *write down* their goals and their considerations and comments in terms of the given criteria as opposed to just thinking about everything.

The third group was not only asked to write down their goals like group 2 but also to *record the actions* they would take (i.e., recording their processes, Q4,).

The fourth group was asked to do everything the third group did with the addition of *sharing their commitments* with a friend (i.e., people, Q3).

The fifth group took the actions of the fourth group further in that each participant in this group sent a written weekly progress report to their weekly accountability partner-friend (thus taking the people, Q3, component of the Synergy Success Cycle to another level).

Let's look at the results of Gail Matthews' goal-setting study. First, and perhaps not surprisingly, the results showed a significant increase in the likelihood of achieving goals for people who wrote them down (groups 2 to 5) versus those who simply thought about them (group 1). The results also showed that 43% of the first group either accomplished their goals or were at least halfway there. Group 4, the participants who shared their goals with other people (Q3), had 63% of participants on track. This demonstrated an almost 20% "bump" by engaging the people component when each participant simply shared their goal with another person. When the group 5 participants not only shared the goal with another person, but also remained in regular contact, giving status updates, an astonishing 76% were on track with their goals.

This is a landmark study in achieving goals. In summary, this study validates the following:

- The power of not only knowing your goals but also recording them
- The power of engaging people in your life
- The power of a clear written action plan with regular accountability with other people included in the plan

Interestingly, I would've liked to have seen in this study a "group 0" that would've included people who would be asked to identify a project they were working on but they would never be asked to articulate in any form their goals with the project. In this way, "group 0" would act as a kind of control group. I can only speculate that a very small percentage of those people would accomplish their project if they lacked a clear goal for their result. You've got to have goals, my friend.

Also, I wonder what would have been the percentage of success if there had've been a group 6. Group 6 would have all the components of the successful fifth group, but also they would create their goals while in a peak state, thus utilizing the extra horsepower proposed by the state-dependent theory. Plus, it would be interesting to learn the results if they re-wrote their goals daily and had mentors in their lives to teach them additional strategies (in addition to their accountability friend/partner). If the fifth group had a 76% success rate, can you imagine the results of this highly engaged group?

Gail Matthews' goal-setting study is probably one of the most foundational validating studies of all the principles that I've outlined in the Synergy Success Cycle. The study directed participants to actively look at all the quadrants from power (Q1) to purpose (Q2) to people (Q3) and to processes (Q4) specifically related to achieving a goal. According to this research, if you follow the Synergy Success Cycle, at the minimum, you place yourself in group 5, where 76% of people achieved their goals. Remember, the framework we are outlining in this book goes beyond the processes outlined in this landmark study, so I predict that when engaging with this framework you will have even better odds than 76% in reaching success!

SMART Goals

A valuable method to help guide you in goal setting is the SMART goal system. SMART is an acronym standing for "specific," "measurable," "attainable," "relevant," and "time-based." Using the SMART goal system allows you to standardize and hone your goals, which sets you up for the greatest likelihood for success.

The S in SMART: S or being "specific" in setting your goals is really important. Most people say, for example, that they want to "be healthy." How are they measuring that? Is it a certain weight or BMI or body fat composition? Is it fitting into a certain dress? The brain needs specificity in order to know how to target its energy.

The M in SMART: M is "measurable," and your health goals also need to be measurable. In order to know you are making progress, you have to find a way to quantify that progress via regular measurements throughout the timeline of achieving your goal.

The A in SMART: A is "attainable," and your SMART goal should be attainable. With "attainable" meaning "not impossible." While I believe that creating attainable goals is good for perpetual motivation and positive reinforcement, I only like to apply the attainability characteristic to my small step goals versus my overall large goals, something I'll outline in the MAGIC goals section of this chapter. In small step goals, you have to have some degree of attainability; otherwise, your brain will ask, "Why bother?"

The R in SMART: R is "relevant." Does your measurable target really matter in the big scheme of the goal? It is important to ask yourself if your goal is relevant to your achieving your ultimate vision. Sometimes we can get stuck on creating a specific goal and spend a lot of energy to obtain it. Once we attain it, we might then realize that the goal that we were striving for was not even relevant to our ultimate vision that we are hoping for. For instance, we can want to lose weight and focus on losing pounds, when, perhaps, losing body fat is more relevant to creating optimal health. Another example: we can want to bulk up at the gym to attain a muscular-looking appearance, but what might be more relevant to our health is to be fully physically functional and perform our daily activities with ease. The question of relevance is a good checks-and-balance system to see if you are on the right track for what you are targeting.

The T in SMART: T is for "time-based," and it is often one of the most overlooked parts of the equation. People work well with deadlines. Creating a timeframe that is specific will help you identify how much time and energy you need to devote to making your SMART goal a reality. Due dates work. Anytime I consult a patient on achieving a specific outcome, I always ask them specifically on what day and even what time they aim to complete the outcome. This creates a line in the sand with a clear due date to hold every party accountable.

I also want to encourage you to learn the art of compressing time. Let me introduce Parkinson's Law. This law discovered that "work expands so as to fill the time available for its completion."[17] Another way of saying this is that whatever amount of time you give a project to complete it, you will more than likely take that full amount of time to complete it. If we created a goal to lose ten pounds in one year, it will probably take one year. However, if we create a goal to lose ten pounds in three months, we can probably accomplish that too. The takeaway is that when creating time-based goals, you want to find the sweet spot for creating an attainable goal in the shortest period of time possible. This will increase your creativity while keeping you focused and avoiding the distractions that having too much time typically allows for.

You definitely want to have SMART goals in all areas of your life, including your health. The brain likes certainty and will use its reticular activating system in helping you achieve those SMART goals. Let's quickly revisit the reticular activating system that we first looked at early on in the book. The reticular activating system is a neural network in your brainstem that filters out unnecessary information and creates focus and alertness to relevant information. Your reticular activating system is at work when you can hear your name in a crowded room or while you are having a conversation with someone in that crowded room. You are able to focus on that conversation while tuning out the other conversations. It is also at work when you experience buying a certain type of vehicle and afterwards you see that type of vehicle commonly on the road whereas previously you never took notice. The ears *hear* and the eyes *see* what the *brain* is looking for. By setting SMART goals, you are essentially activating your reticular activating system to focus on situations, events, and relationships to help you achieve your goals.

Many top leaders also talk about the importance of frequently reviewing goals. CEO and author Grant Cardone revealed that he writes down his goals twice a day. The first time when waking up in the morning as a means to turn on his reticular activating system. The second time right before going to bed as a way to have these goals work in his subconscious while sleeping. I think this is a great strategy because it involves kinesthetically writing down the goals, seeing them on paper visually, and then reading them aloud after writing them. All of which will further reinforce the power of the reticular activating system and its magnetic force in helping you achieve your goals. Again, putting yourself in a positive state of mind (i.e., as given in the state-dependent theory) while writing your goals, for example, by listening to inspiring music or utilizing your sense of smell with an invigorating essential oil, can take this goal setting to another level.

From SMART to MAGIC

I like SMART goals. They serve as solid incremental steps in helping us to achieve our goals. Rarely, though, will we achieve something of true greatness, true transformation, if we are only setting goals that are SMART. Sometimes we have to be unreasonable in life and think significantly greater—and go way, way beyond the "attainable" and "realistic." That is where the real magic happens and that is where the true innovators who seek out an exceptional quality of life dare to live. The greats who have changed society—from civil rights to the technology we enjoy today—did more than simply create SMART goals.

To harness the importance of setting truly spectacular goals I created a new acronym called **MAGIC goals**. These are your big vision goals. In Jim Collins' book *Good to Great*, he calls them BHAG goals, with BHAG standing for "big hairy audacious goals." MAGIC goals stand for giant goals that are:

- Measurable
- Attractive
- Giant
- Inspiring
- Creative

For MAGIC to happen you want to let your mind run free and explore what is possible! This is where you want to not get constrained by "how" you are going to do something, but rather dare to dream up the big "what" that you really want. Our logical brain limits us when creating big goals. When we create a big goal, our logical brain taps us on the shoulder and says, "Okay, you, exactly how are you going to do this?" This immediately stops the flow in the process of creating big goals. Do not do this. Do not get stuck in the "how" of the attainment of MAGIC goals. Get more focused on the big "what" that you want to accomplish.

Because of the reticular activating system, making these MAGIC goals **measurable** is still critical. Saying you want to be a millionaire versus you want to have a net worth of a 100 million dollars by a certain age are two very different statements for the brain to process. Running a 5K as a SMART health goal is nice, but running a marathon is sexy. The level of training, both physically and emotionally, involved in completing a marathon is completely different than a 5K. With marathon training, you need a detailed running schedule, the support of others, significant time commitments, and a more regimented meal plan. In order to do something magical like completing a marathon, you have to become someone potentially completely different than who you once were. You know you are striving for a MAGIC goal when you are transforming into a new person. You know you are in the pursuit of MAGIC goals when friends who have not seen you in a while feel that your presence is different.

Another MAGIC goal that can be transformative is when a person decides to get off lifestyle medications. Lifestyle medications are those medicines that once your doctor prescribes them, it is rare to stop taking them, and they become part of the person's life. These medications range from high blood pressure pills, medication for diabetes, over-the-counter pain medicine (a big no-no), sleep medication, and psychotropic drugs for anxiety, depression, and attention.

After being on these medications for years, it is not a simple task to stop using them, but it is possible. First, I must disclose that I am not your doctor, nor am I a medical doctor, so do not alter your medications without working with the doctor who prescribed them. But, I do recommend that if you decide to create a MAGIC goal to become independent of your lifestyle medication, once you clearly and intentionally express your deep desire to get off of them, then you could ask your doctor if they have had success in helping others get off of the same medication and then have the doctor clearly outline a strategy to do so. If your doctor is not willing to actively engage in helping you achieve this goal, then you may want to see if they have a colleague who will. (We will talk about this in more detail in the people quadrant, specifically, getting the right people on your health team). Remember, you have to take personal responsibility and your doctors work for you in helping you get to your health goals.

Your MAGIC goal needs to be super **attractive** to you. When you think about the attainment of this MAGIC goal, you are allured, captivated, enticed, and fascinated by it so much so that you are willing to do whatever it takes to achieve it. When you are attracted to it, it will serve as a mental magnet in your life. MAGIC goals need to be giant! In his book *The 10X Rule*, Grant Cardone states that one of biggest mistakes people make when goal setting is that their goals are way too small. He recommends taking your goals and multiplying them by ten, thus the title of his book *The 10X Rule*!

Make your measurable MAGIC goal so GIANT that you are uncomfortable. If you are comfortable with the goal, then it is an attainable goal and, therefore, does not qualify as a MAGIC goal (but rather as a SMART goal). Go wild here. You can either put your energy into the reasons why something can or cannot happen, or be unreasonable and set your bar high. Even if you don't reach your MAGIC goal and fall short, you still probably will have achieved far more than you thought was ever possible.

Your MAGIC goal needs to be **inspiring**. Inspiring means bringing "in" the spirit. Inspiring goals create the heart of your goal, one that has both the emotional juice that an attractive goal provides and also the spiritual energy you will bring within yourself to help make it a priority to every cell in your body. Attractive goals work with the mind, and inspiring goals work with the spirit.

MAGIC goals elicit the **creative** process. Once our brain is targeted on the specific measurable giant goal that we want to achieve, our mind is attracted to its attainment. And the spirit is inspired. All of this primes the pump for our creative processes to go to work. Keep your full self attuned to the MAGIC goals, and you will start to see creative ways for their fulfillment. This is not some mystical method, but again it is using the power of your own physiology, your own reticular activating system. This is also coupled with the fact that we are all made of atoms and energy.

When we create MAGIC goals, we start to resonate and identify with them. I believe that our reticular activating system acts as our filter to seek the creative solutions in the environment, and our energy attracts those people who are on a similar path as us. Essentially our commitment and emotional and spiritual proximity with our MAGIC goals work together to send an intentional energy out to the world. All the while, other people's reticular activating systems are looking for environments and stimuli that match their filters.

Compounding and Leveraging

I bet most of you have never thought about making goals beyond ten years out. I have learned that the most successful achievers think much further into the future and have a greater appreciation of the time and effort it takes to achieve a truly MAGIC goal. They also understand the power of compounding. People tend to think about the power of compounding in reference to the idea of compounding interest. The power of compounding interest reveals that as time goes on, investments, where the interest payments are reinvested, create exponential growth.

The power of compounding also applies when you reinvest the growth, knowledge, and skills over time in the obtainment of your ultimate goal. Knowledge and skills are an incredible resource that often can stay with us throughout our life. This is why education and experience are such incredible assets. A chiropractor who has been caring for patients for 20 years has an entirely different skill set capability than a recent graduate because of the compounding of knowledge and experience. The experienced chiropractor is dramatically more effective at helping the patient reach their health goal. When you are achieving your health goals, do not discount the education, knowledge, and skills you have learned throughout your life. Leverage that experience to propel yourself to the next level. Leverage the past health victories to serve as validation to increase your self-confidence and power to take your health to the next level.

Through this first half of the Synergy Success Cycle via the inner work of quadrants 1 and 2, power and purpose, we have inched our way to the second part, the outer expression. Don't, however, underestimate the power of those inches! As golfing legend Arnold Palmer stated, "Golf is a game of inches. The most important are the six inches between your ears." Although golf, life, and the pursuit of achieving our ultimate health involve a significant amount of technical skills, mastered over time, we must first master our mind. Mastering the elements of your power and harnessing your purpose are the first two parts of the Synergy Success Cycle framework. However, only knowing who you are, what you want, and why you want it will not get the health you are seeking. Manifesting and expressing our true health potential only occurs when we engage the second half of the Synergy Success Cycle—the outer expression: quadrants 3 and 4. Section 2 of the Synergy Success Cycle involves the people in our lives (Q3) and the processes and actions we must take to make our dreams a reality (Q4).

Synergy Action Steps

1. Looking at your vision that you have started to create in the previous chapter, what is a MAGIC goal related to your health?
2. Is it GIANT enough? Do you need to 10X your MAGIC goal like Grant Cardone would say?
3. What are some SMART goals that you need to create to get you closer towards your MAGIC goal over the next month, next 90 days, next year, and next five, ten, 20, or 40 years?

QUADRANT 3 PEOPLE AND QUADRANT 4 PROCESS

Congratulations! You are halfway through the Synergy Success Cycle. For most of us, the inner work is the most challenging. Working within our own mind is much more complex than what we can see right before our eyes. The inner work is also where we often get stuck and quit before we take any meaningful action. Remembering your power (Q1) and purpose (Q2) will get you through your action plan (Q4). But to create anything meaningful, truly impactful we have to have the right people around us (Q3) and we have to have a plan backed up by action (Q4). That is where the second part of the Synergy Success Cycle enters the game. We will answer the question of "Who else?" in the people quadrant (Q4) and "How does it get done?" in the process quadrant (Q4).

The stronger and more developed the first part of the cycle, the inner work (Q1 and Q2), like a magnet, the more you will attract the right people in your life who are consistent with your purpose, vision, and goals. The first part of the Synergy Success Cycle is, therefore, about recognizing your strengths and values and then crystalizing your purpose, vision, and goals to create such an internal force within yourself that you can move mountains. Moving forward, you create momentum by exploring the various groups of people (Q3) you need in your life to make magical things happen to your health. The following chapters, dedicated to the third quadrant, will cover:

- Chapter 14: the people who are your health leaders and role models
- Chapter 15: the people on your team and your accountability partners
- Chapter 16: the people you serve and care for

And so we launch into the third quadrant, starting with the people who are your role models.

Q3 PEOPLE—YOUR HEALTH LEADERS AND ROLE MODELS

One of the greatest values of mentors is the ability to see what others cannot see and to help them navigate a course to their destination.

—John Maxwell

Before asking how to do something—which is the fourth and final quadrant on process—it is important to first ask *who* has done it before. This brings us to the third quadrant in the Synergy Success Cycle—people. Recognizing the people in and around you is the first step in externally manifesting your ultimate vision for all areas of your life, including your health. When I refer to the people around you who have done it before, I'm pointing to mentors, coaches, teachers, and leaders who do or could serve as your role models. Yes, it is even crucial to have role models to achieve your optimal health!

Role models allow us to see the behaviors and actions we desire for ourselves already at play in people who have obtained success in a given area. Role models come in many forms. Some people are lucky (or intentional enough) to have mentors who guide and encourage them along the way. A mentor is a trusted advisor, someone who has "been there and done that," and has a lot of life experience in a particular area. Not only do they have the knowledge combined with the experience, they have a teaching spirit and are willing to share their wisdom along the way.

Mentors are more precious and rarer than the finest cars or jewels. Sadly, too few of us seek out and cultivate these relationships. I believe this occurs because many people's level of personal power, as discussed in the first quadrant, limits their self-identity. They see someone who is achieving success and say to themselves, "I can't do that," "Why would that person want to teach and advise me?" or "Who am I to be worthy of this person's guidance?" Unfortunately, people's limiting beliefs and limiting self-concepts are the very reason many don't have a vast network of mentors.

You need to know that God has you here for a purpose. A life with purpose is not reserved to just a select few but for all of us. There are people out there who get a high level of personal fulfillment by helping others gain the success they have already gained. Most successful people recognize that their success was not achieved by themselves alone but because others guided them. Mentorship is a way of paying it back.

Mentors gain pleasure from coaching and teaching. They get excited when they hear aspiring individuals share their passion and their purpose about a subject that they know a lot about. This is why it is so important for you to get clear on your purpose, vision, and goals, and share them with those around you. You never know how it could inspire those in your circle to better define their own purpose, vision, and goals. You never know who they know that they can connect you with to help make your dreams a reality.

Your dreams and desires, when given the right attention and energy, will literally seek out ways to be expressed. Like the famous scene in the movie *Jerry McGuire* when Cuba Gooding says, "Show me the money!" He is putting out to the world an intention, with high energy, about what he desires. I remember when I started my chiropractic practice and I had no patient base, I would drive my car listening to upbeat, inspiring music and yell, "Show me the patients!" Now, I can't confirm if that was the secret, but we've never had a new patient problem in our 18-year history!

I also recall one of our team huddles, before we opened for patient care, when I asked the team to describe details about a potential future new patient that would reach out to us that very day to secure an open time slot we had later that day in our schedule. Mind you, this person had not called us yet. One of the front desk patient coordinators enthusiastically stated that it would be a young lady. I asked her to describe the kind of car the young lady drove. My team member looked at me oddly but played along, answering that the young lady would be driving a jeep. Going deeper in setting the intention, I asked her to provide the jeep's color. Still puzzled by my questions, but playing along, she stated it would be orange. To be honest, I had doubts, I mean, how many young women do you know who drive jeeps that are orange? I went with it though, and the team agreed that later that day we were going to see a young lady who drove an orange jeep.

Later that day, we did have someone call in and come in for that opening. To my astonishment, it was a free-spirited young lady about 24 years old. I asked her, out of curiosity, about the kind of car she drove, and she told me, a jeep! I almost fell over! The color of her jeep was yellow, but pretty darn close! The team was shocked and amazed. The takeaway: you never know how what you put out there in the universe with energy and intention will show up in your life. The more you speak, envision, and write about what you want, the more you will attract the right people (Q3), including those precious mentors who will take your life—and your health—to the next level.

Besides mentors, coaches can help bring out your strengths. Mentors often teach you by sharing stories of their experiences, so you can learn principles and lessons. Coaches are different in that they dig into you and ask questions. They discover more about what you are currently doing and where you want to go. They also can key in on how you are thinking about the results you are trying to achieve. They are learning your "modus operandi" or the code of how you operate. While not all mentors are coaches, most coaches are mentors because they often have extensive experience. Again, true coaches are rare jewels that we never forget.

As a chiropractor, I was extremely blessed to have such an impactful role model in my life at a very young age. Dr. Elliott, whom I've already mentioned, was the single most important element in helping me create (Q4) a top chiropractic practice and provide me with a compelling purpose (Q2). Having Dr. Elliott as a role model, mentor, and coach (Q2) enabled me to serve almost twenty thousand people, deliver over a quarter of a million adjustments, and produce high levels of personal and professional success for myself and my team.

When I've spoken at the University of Central Florida, for several of its colleges, including its colleges of medicine, business, engineering, and health and public affairs, I always ask who in the audience has a mentor. Statistically about 5% of the people raise their hands. Often, these people found their mentors as impressionable young people often in a time of need, which is very similar to my own story when, as a young boy with scoliosis, I found Dr. Elliot. It's funny how many of us have come to know our mentors as a result of dealing with a perceived negative issue. Yet those of us with mentors to help us traverse these perceived negative situations are the ones who have the greatest advantage, in my opinion. If you want to expand the quality of your life in a particular area, for example, in terms of your health, and you do not have role models, I believe that you are at the greatest disadvantage. Role models teach you the best processes, the fourth quadrant of the Synergy Success Cycle, the processes that propelled them to high levels of achievement.

Often, I get asked, "How do I find a mentor? How do I find a mentor, trusted counselor, or guide who is willing to share their experiences, successes, and failures to help me along the way?" Here are some rules to creating a mentor relationship that I have found valuable:

Be open and receptive.

You have to be coachable. "Coachable" means that you're willing to take instruction, guidance, and constructive criticism in a positive light. When someone wants help from somebody and they give it to them, it is oftentimes considered coaching. When someone is not really open to help or is not coachable, they view the help as negative criticism. A lot of people say they're coachable, but the truth is that few people are coachable. That is because many people hold on to a belief system, which may be limited in a particular area, so they are blind to the things they are trying to learn about. This also makes them resistant to being coached on better strategies.

A mentor should not be in your chain of command.

It is hard for a mentor to be your boss. You want to be able to have honest, open conversations about not only your strengths, but concerns about your weaknesses. If you are trying to do this with your boss, it may be hard for you to share your worries because you don't want to look bad or inept. Also, it is hard for a mentor, as a boss, to fully give you their opinion or assessment if you are their employee for fear or concern about damaging the employer/employee relationship. Because there are many social norms today around political correctness, it is hard for a person in a position of power in an organization to tell you what you need to hear and say it in a way that will make an impact on you while at the same time protecting the organization. For these reasons, I suggest that you find a mentor that is out of your chain of command, so neither of you will have to worry or be constrained.

You need to become noticed for personal mentorship.

If you want someone of value to help you, you need to emerge from obscurity. Because of our own limiting beliefs and our lower self-identity in a particular area of life, that we are seeking to improve, we can struggle with the question of "Who am I to be worthy of having a meaningful mentor relationship with this person who is highly successful and gifted in this area?" This thought pattern will restrict us from stepping up, taking initiative, and becoming noticed. You must realize that every successful person in an area started where you are. When you come to them in a humble, but excited way, then you will remind them of where they once were at the start of their journey to success. Be creative and persistent in making yourself noticed.

Once you create this relationship, find ways to add value to the relationship, so it is not all one-sided.

At the beginning, many of us cannot afford to buy professional coaching, consulting, or mentorship. Instead, we have to buy it with our time, energy, and sweat equity. I learned some of the best practice systems in chiropractic through my Thursday mentorship sessions with Dr. Dan. As already discussed, I worked for Dr. Dan at his thriving chiropractic practice on my day off without any financial compensation. I did whatever he wanted me to do for the practice, including helping him with patients, preparing charts, and analyzing X-rays. All these tasks would have normally paid me thousands of dollars but working for him for free gave me million-dollar strategies. I tell students that it is better to work for somebody for free who will mentor you versus working for them for $10 an hour. There is a societal norm to reciprocate. If I pay you $10 an hour to do a job, then I do not feel the need to reciprocate because my payment was the reciprocation for the work you did. If, however, you work for me for free, I have a societal and moral obligation to give back to you something of value. This will often be in the form of mentorship, guidance, knowledge, or wisdom.

Your mentors may or may not know you.

Don't limit your thinking that you have to have a personal relationship with a mentor to understand and learn lessons as well as best practices. With the abundant amount of information posted on the internet, you can really go deep in understanding a person's thought processes, lessons, and best practices by becoming their student. Many thought leaders have podcasts, extensive YouTube channels, books, online courses, and live events. Some of my best role models have never met me. I've listened to countless hours of John Maxwell on leadership. I shook the hand of, and took a picture with, Grant Cardone for a total of ten seconds of face-to-face contact, yet I have listened to hundreds of hours of his information. My only personal experience with Tony Robbins was 20 seconds of conversation together while I was walking next to him on our way to the fire walk experience at one of his seminars, yet I have studied his concepts for several decades. Brian Tracy is a friend who does not know me. Stephen Covey and I, unfortunately before his passing, never met. Michael Gerber and I never had lunch or coffee. Yet all these people have been pivotal mentors in my life and personal development journey.

Paying for coaching or consulting is a worthy investment.

Many leaders have invested decades of their life and countless hours of trial and error and refinement to get to where they are. The fact that they are thought leaders and successful inherently makes them in demand for people seeking to achieve the same results. Mentoring a person one-on-one is time-consuming, and successful people know that their time is their greatest asset and has a huge value. Mentors seeing the need to share their information combined with a desire to help others will often create programs and events—live or online, intensive workshops, or mastermind groups—for you to gain their knowledge. This can result in a relationship where you must invest financially.

When starting mentorship with a thought leader, an inexpensive way to create this relationship is to buy and read one of their books. For about $20 you can gain well-thought-out, well-composed concepts to help guide you along the way. The next level can be investing in an online course. For several hundreds of dollars you can go deeper, where the creator of the curriculum can guide you and help you increase your understanding of the concepts and map out how they apply specifically to you.

Again, I am offering this type of mentorship experience with my online Synergy Life University. Visit www.The SynergyLife.com to learn more about the Synergy Life University. This type of deeper learning is a powerful and fantastic means to help you grasp the concepts better AND guide you to create action plans. The next level could be attending a live event for several thousands of dollars where now you are in the company and presence of thought leaders and others who probably share similar interests and passions. These seminars could provide brief opportunities to interact with your mentors.

Yet another level can be where you invest a significantly greater amount of money to have either group or one-on-one coaching with your mentor. I have always been willing to invest in coaching and consulting relationships in my professional career because I always felt the inherent cost of making mistakes and the increased time it would take to do it on my own was far more costly than the investment in learning best practices from a coach. In regards to my health, by having a personal trainer, cook, and chiropractor in my life, I am learning better strategies to help my physical health as well as having the accountability to keep me on track.

Your Team of Doctors and Healthcare Providers: Advisors and Role Models

When you think of your doctors, do you consider them as mentors or role models in your health? Are they someone you just see to help you get through an illness, or are they truly an inspirational mentor, leader, or coach that inspires you to take yourself to the next level? When looking at assembling your clinical team of professionals to help take your health to the next level, I encourage you to answer these questions:

- *Do I have all the necessary doctors to support and protect my overall health? Are their certain doctors that I need to add to my personal healthcare team? Is there an area of my health that I have been neglecting or ignoring that I need to engage a specialist to help me work on with more focus?*
- *Do my healthcare providers align with my personal health values and viewpoint? If I value preventative care and they*

only engage to help me in a reactionary manner, is that really the right doctor for me? What if I value a more natural approach and their only solution is artificial drugs, is there a disconnect? What are the viewpoints of my doctors on the other types of healthcare providers that I personally value? Do they refer to, and are they willing to work with, the type of providers that I value?

These are not only important philosophical questions, but also very practical questions. You want a team that will work together. You want a team that will work for you. I think patients forget that they have choices in who they select to be part of their healthcare team. I think patients forget that they pay their doctors for their education, experience, knowledge, and training, BUT that the doctors work for them. A doctor is of little value if there is not a patient to serve.

- *Have you had a conversation with your healthcare team to let them know what your health values are? Have they asked and do they seem interested?*

Take the time to explore the Targeted Health Values List laid out in chapter 7 and discuss it with your health team. Create some healthy dialogue like, "Dr. Jones, I really respect all of your knowledge and training that you have gained to serve so many patients as a wonderful doctor. Since I have so much respect for you, I wanted to share my own health values, so we can be on the same page in helping ensure that my health plan is heading in the right direction. Is that okay with you?" Then share your values.

A good doctor will be excited that you are taking responsibility for your health and will listen. Ask them if their strategies align with your values and viewpoint. If they do, great. If they do not, then have the courage to ask your doctor if they know another doctor that may be better suited to care for you. Although this may seem confrontative, this doctor will respect you. Plus, once you start taking a more active role in your health and become more vocal, then if your values conflict with their approach, they probably won't want to deal with you anyway. They would rather treat patients who agree with their approach, so it really is best for everyone. You are doing yourself and them the best service by having these crucial conversations.

- *Besides traditional medical doctors, what other experts in health do you want or need to add to your team?*

Chiropractors are considered by many still as alternative healthcare providers. Chiropractors that are more "principled" or "corrective" are still focused on the essence of what chiropractic was founded on. Chiropractic was not designed to be for the treatment of disease or symptoms. Chiropractic was not designed as pain management either. Although chiropractic is a wonderful, natural, drug-free, surgery-free healthcare approach to helping reduce pain, that was not the original intent.

Chiropractors, in essence, treat the spine because we know that pressure on the nervous system can affect so many health issues in the body. A chiropractor's role is to locate, detect, and correct misalignments in the spine that cause pressure or interference to the nervous system. The resulting pressure to the nervous system can not only cause pain, early degeneration to the spine discs, and tightened muscles, but also lead to a host of organ issues. It can cause breathing issues, digestive issues, cardiac issues, and immune issues. Now to be clear, not all these conditions are caused by nerve interference, but this interference, if present, can cause a person's body to malfunction. In my professional opinion, most everyone can benefit from chiropractic care as a means of spinal "hygiene" but also nerve system protection.

Besides chiropractors, it is important to have on your health-care team other holistic doctors and providers, such as acupuncturists, mental health counselors, hypnotherapists, massage therapists, personal trainers, yoga and Pilates instructors, and experts in nutrition and exercise. Of course, you cannot forget the importance of regular dental checkups with your dentist as well as the benefits of orthodontic care. There are a lot of other health benefits people don't often associate with proper dental hygiene including cardiovascular health.

Acupuncturists can provide an avenue to help the energy in your body flow properly. One of my college professors explained that chiropractors work on the fuse box and the power switches that control the flow of electricity in your body. Acupuncturists work on the quality of that electricity.

We also know that motion is life. If we look at a living cell in a microscope and see no motion, we know that cell is dead. If you don't use things in life, you lose them. This makes exercise and meaningful movement critical. Having an expert help you in getting crisp motion of your joints is critical to maintaining a healthy structure, and that movement literally feeds your brain as well. Do you need to engage a physical or occupational therapist to rehabilitate an old injury or a repetitive strain injury that has been neglected? Do you need to hire an experienced personal trainer to help you optimize your muscle system, maintain functional movement, or build strength? As we age, we have to work harder than before just to keep the same health results. For this, look to chiropractic, personal trainers, physical therapists, massage therapists, occupational therapists, yoga and Pilates instructors, or occupational therapists.

Psychologists and counselors offer therapy without the use of prescription medication while psychiatrists tend to prescribe medication. If your past is holding you back emotionally, then you should be adding these important experts to your team. Be sure too that the type of emotional expert you select matches your value preference. This is really important here.

Coaches, as we have described earlier, also help support you emotionally but are not focused on healing past wounds—that is the realm of the psychologist, counselor, and psychiatrist. Coaches are experts at helping you become aware of who you are, the goals you want to create, and they serve as an accountability partner to help you reach your goals. *The Synergy Health Solution* essentially is a coaching book to guide you through the Synergy Success Cycle to help you achieve your best health and life.

Synergy Action Steps

1. Who are your current role models in your life as it pertains to your health?
2. Which ones do you have personal relationships with?
3. Which role models are ones that you study from a distance (online or in books)?
4. Who are new potential role models that you need to engage with in regards to your health?
5. Examine your healthcare advisory team. Who is on your healthcare advisory team? When looking at each member of your team, who is missing? Who needs to be replaced? Who do you need to have a consultation with to refocus them back to your goals?

CHAPTER 15

Q3 PEOPLE—TEAM MEMBERS AND ACCOUNTABILITY PARTNERS

Coming together is a beginning. Keeping together is progress. Working together is success.

—Henry Ford

Big visions require a lot of hands on deck. In order to achieve any significant accomplishment, you should have people on your team, meaning a team that helps you execute your vision and that supports you.

In the chiropractic industry, the majority of offices consist of one doctor and two staff members. In addition, the doctor is handling the company finances as well as all the marketing and community relations. The doctor is also doing everything in regard to patient care. They are doing the intakes, history, examination, case management, adjustments, therapies, X-rays, and all the charts and notes. The doctor is doing it all. Most doctors try to keep their business overhead low, which seems appealing at first glance. The reality, though, is that doing all this themselves ends up burning the doctor out, shortening their career, and limiting the impact that they can make on their community.

Sadly, most small businesses also consist of one person doing all the jobs, roles, and responsibilities. We do this because we think we are saving money and that no one can do the work that we do just like we do it. In reality, if you're going to make a big impact in an area of your life, you are going to need people on your team that will support you and help you execute your vision. You simply can't do it all.

As we talked about in the power quadrant (Q1), we all are gifted with unique strengths, talents, and abilities. It is impossible for you to be completely successful and maximize your potential with solely your own unique strengths, talents, and abilities. You are going to need people added to your team that complement you and provide strengths to fill in the gaps. Many visionaries are not very good at day-to-day management. And day-to-day managers are not good at seeing the big picture. We need both—people who are task-oriented and others who are people-oriented. We need those who are fast-paced to keep everything moving and those who will methodically slow things down to ensure all the steps are being completed and nothing is missed.

When I talk to small business owners, many relate that the hardest thing to handle in their business is not necessarily their particular product or service. They typically have developed good systems to deliver the product or service in a predictable manner. The challenge for most small business owners is finding, onboarding, and developing the right people for their team in the right positions. I know for me personally this has been the greatest challenge because it is difficult to find people that match my standard and work ethic and who align with the values and vision of the practice. This is something that I perpetually work on and I know that I can always get better at.

Similarly, when looking at our health, we need to carefully select the right team members to support us in our health vision and goals. As you likely discovered in the previous chapter, your healthcare team probably has some deficiencies.

The first thing you want to do is make sure that you are clear on your values for your health and your viewpoint, both of which we covered in chapter 7. If you value a non-drug approach and a vitalistic point of view that sees the body as designed to heal and we just need to remove the interferences, then you should determine if your team supports this point of view. If you prefer a non-drug approach first and the first thing your doctor does is write a prescription, then you may have the wrong person on your team. They could be the right person, provided you express your preference and they honor that preference as well as demonstrate the ability to provide some alternative solutions outside of a prescription pad.

Again, I'm not saying that all drugs are bad and that they don't have a place in your healthcare framework. I'm asking you to determine where that fits in your framework and in what sequence. For me, it is (1) natural healing methods and chiropractic first, then (2) more aggressive approaches, such as drugs, and only as a last resort (3), surgery. What is your sequence? Does your current team provide a framework that supports your sequence, approach, and philosophy?

Also, realize that people take medications in two ways. One is for an acute episode, such as a cold or an infection. This is typically a dose of medication for a short period of time. The second type of medication protocol is chronic disease management, which we earlier called lifestyle medication. This medication strategy involves taking medication for life. This might be cholesterol medication, thyroid medication, diabetes medication, or psychotropic drugs.

What about pain medication? Do you think it should be taken episodically for just a short period of time, or is it something that is intermittently taken for decades? How have you been managing your pain? What about antianxiety or antidepressant medication? Is that something taken to help you through a particular episode of an impactful life event? Or is it something that is taken for the rest of your life? I am not here to give you medical advice about your prescriptions, but the questions do beg for some contemplation to see what matches your philosophy of health and your ideal approach as well as the support or opposition you will get from the doctor leading your care.

Your Two Essential Teams

Another way of looking at your heath team is to have two health provider teams. One is a team that focuses on your health and the protection of it, which I call your "health" team. The other is a team of doctors to help in an emergency when you are sick, called your "sick" team. Most people unfortunately only have the sick team of doctors, yet they think they have a complete healthcare team. Your health team should be a team that is designed to support and enhance the optimal *function* of your body, mind, and spirit, the true definition of health as defined earlier. When things get too out of hand or if a trauma occurs, you need to call on your other team.

The sick team will help you manage any crisis, disease or condition that may have slipped through the cracks of you and your health team. The "sick" care team has an arsenal of pharmaceutical drugs, intensive treatments, and invasive surgeries, which they have expertly trained on. Again, they should be your last warriors on the defense to help keep you alive in critical times of poor health. Do you have both of these teams set up? You should.

What does a health team look like? First of all, your healthcare team doesn't necessarily have to include only doctors. I consider my personal trainer as part of my healthcare team. He helps to support my musculoskeletal system as well as integrate the various muscle groups to function in an optimal way to support the activities that I do, as well as my posture.

My wife is part of my health team in many ways. Besides being supportive and positive, she is also strategic. She orders boxed meals that are shipped to our house from various companies. The boxes come with fresh organic foods that have been cleaned and portioned, and they include all the spices and condiments needed to prepare them along with a recipe card. This provides us an alternative to going out to dinner, which would put us in less control of what we are eating and how it is prepared. I consider these health food alternative companies as part of my health team.

One trick that my wife did is definitely worth sharing. Now this is a process (Q4) health hack, but it is worth giving you a preview of how getting the right people can make processes easier. In the beginning, we had babysitters come and play with our children and watch them while my wife was in the kitchen cooking and running around doing the laundry as well as light cleaning. We then had an epiphany. We decided to switch that approach. We created a scenario where the babysitter changed roles to a mother's helper, meaning she prepares the meals that are delivered from these companies, does the laundry, and does light cleaning while we get to engage and connect more with our children. For many parents, 4 pm to 7 pm are the witching hours. They are running around, getting the kids to do their homework, preparing meals, cleaning the house, all while being exhausted from a day at work. This switching of roles, from babysitter to mother's helper, eradicates the witching hour.

I suggest checking out websites such as www.Care.com to find a helper that is a local high school person who maybe has younger siblings and a desire to help. It's not only good for your family, it does a whole lot to teach the young person you hire important lessons in responsibility.

Your gym or fitness studio is part of your health team. The people who run the group exercise classes are part of your team. Consider making these places and the people who run them part of your health team versus just a place that you go to. A simple mindset shift that they are part of your team will increase your connection and engagement to the process (Q4) and to them (Q3). Don't forget about focused fitness facilities, such as yoga or Pilates studios, or other functional fitness training studios that incorporate high intensity interval training (also called HIIT) with heart rate monitors.

Where are you getting your nutritional advice? We all know that diet and exercise are the two areas that everybody speaks about when we talk about "getting healthy." Are you eating solely based on when your blood sugar drops and you seek out the closest and fastest convenience food? Or do you have some level of meal planning as well as access to healthy small snacks to fuel you throughout the day? People tend to get their health advice on eating from sources such as television programs, social media, advertising, friends, books, videos, magazines, and podcasts. This book is not designed to go deep into nutrition, but it is important that you are carefully selecting who you are getting your nutritional advice from and that you have a system to monitor if that approach is working well for you.

Obviously as a chiropractor, I believe that everyone should have a chiropractor on their health team. Studies show that somewhere between 10% to 20% of people utilize chiropractic. Unfortunately, the general public has not been trained properly as to the role of chiropractic and the importance of having it as part of their health team. Chiropractors are trained to the same level as medical doctors in terms of classroom hours. Chiropractors must attend undergraduate college and take similar prerequisite courses, such as chemistry, physics, and biology. Rather than attending medical school, they attend chiropractic school. This is no different than a dentist going to dental school or a podiatrist going to podiatrist school. My chiropractic college was ten trimesters. A typical undergraduate class schedule is somewhere between 12 to 15 hours of classroom time per week over four years. Chiropractic college consists of 30 to 35 hours of classroom time per week followed by an additional 20 to 30 hours of study weekly. The training was rigorous and intensive. The general public does not fully appreciate the sacrifice their doctors make in preparing themselves to take care of patients.

Rather than having extensive hours on pharmacology or surgery, a chiropractor spends those hours in learning how to properly and safely manipulate and adjust the spine as well as other joints. They also learn other physiotherapy techniques to support the neuromusculoskeletal system. Throughout the chiropractic training, a US chiropractor must complete a series of four national board examinations as well as individual state requirements. Chiropractors do not have residencies in hospitals like their medical counterparts simply because they are not often involved in the hospital-based, sick-care crisis model. Rather, most chiropractors invest a few years working as an associate in an established chiropractic practice serving a community. This provides them with the opportunity to learn and develop their skills very much like a medical doctor does in a hospital.

Now that we talked about the training of a chiropractor, let's talk about what they do and their ideal role as part of your health team. Chiropractic is a philosophy, science, and art. The philosophy of chiropractic is one that recognizes that the nervous system controls and coordinates all body functions and is essentially the master system. Your nervous system is the first system to be created as you are developing inside your mother's womb. The spinal cord starts to take shape after 18 days of conception.

The second principle of chiropractic is that the body is designed to heal. If you cut your finger, you do not have to intentionally think about all the activities required to help that area heal and repair. The body, with its own intelligence that we talked about earlier, will send white blood cells to the area to contain and destroy any foreign bacteria to prevent infection, it will supply the area with fresh red blood cells, and it will orchestrate the perfect sequence of cells to repair, close, and heal the cut. Your body is designed to go towards health and not disease. The chiropractor's role then is not to "treat" the body but rather to remove the nerve interference preventing the body from healing. Rather than chasing a symptom and treating it with a medication, to stop the symptom, a chiropractor typically adjusts the spine to take pressure off of the nervous system to allow the body to properly communicate with itself and heal the way it was inherently designed to do.

In addition, chiropractic understands that the human frame should have an optimal position including a strong upright posture. One force that we cannot make go away is gravity. If our body is out of alignment, gravitational forces cause the joints, ligaments, and discs to load unevenly. There are well-documented effects to the spine that can cause it to break down prematurely in key areas of pressure. The problem is these areas of pressure result in increased bone formation, commonly called arthritis, which then can trap the exiting nerves that go to muscles and organs in the body. Just like teeth can decay without proper care, the spine can decay prematurely without proper care.

Those who are interested in my chiropractic practice in Oviedo, Florida can visit my website at www.SynergyOviedo.com.

Dentists have done a phenomenal job at teaching the concept of dental hygiene. The chiropractic profession, sadly, has done a much poorer job at teaching the concept of spinal hygiene. And spinal hygiene is worsening in modern times with the increased use of mobile devices and laptops. Our children have their necks in an abnormally flexed position for prolonged periods of time, which creates significantly worse problems to spinal health at significantly younger ages. Also, they are carrying heavy loads on their spines with backpacks that are too heavy. Children are playing competitive sports at younger and younger ages, and any lingering injury, not properly handled, can produce a significant long-term health consequence during a rapid growth spurt. For these reasons, I believe that you should have a chiropractor on your health team to support the structure of your spine and entire physical frame.

Health Accountability Partners

Gail Matthews' research around goal setting that we discussed in chapter 13 shows clear and compelling evidence about the value of an accountability partner. There is no doubt in my mind that your success can be increased by having the right accountability partner on your health team. As already mentioned, I struggle with consistently working out because I do so early in the morning as that is the best time for my schedule. When that alarm clock went off at 4:25 am and I was going to a spin class with no accountability partner, it was very easy for me to turn off the alarm and justify to myself that the extra sleep was more important. Since my trainer comes to my house at 4:50 am, I know that I must be up, ready, and willing to do the workload. I am always more consistent when I have an accountability partner, especially when I am paying for it! If I was to go back to the spin class, I would ensure that I have an accountability partner who also attended the class. Ideally, it would be great if the person running the class created an opportunity for people to have accountability partners established formally.

Consider having multiple accountability partners for each area of your life. Who is your accountability partner in the area of your exercise and fitness? Who is your accountability partner when it comes to your nutrition? Who is your accountability partner to help you with your mental health? Who is your accountability partner to help you with your overall physical body?

Is your significant other part of your accountability team, or are they either disengaged or not aligned with your vision and goals? This can be a tough situation if your spouse is at odds with your vision and goals. Situations like this involve the courage to have crucial conversations and mutual respect to honor each other's values and viewpoints. Oftentimes your spouse's motivation to improve a particular area may not occur at the same time or season as yours. That is part of life. That is part of a relationship. No two people are exactly alike or are focusing on the exact same things at the exact same time. But through mutual respect, understanding, and appreciation hopefully your partner will at least support you in your endeavors.

If your significant other is your accountability partner in some aspect of your health, you are blessed. If they are not, then you need to seek an accountability partner outside of the relationship while at the same time continue to find ways to support and nurture your significant other.

Investing in Your Health

There always seem to be more expenses than money coming in. Certainly, it is wise to look at where you are spending your money. Many of us have families to support and debts to pay down. However, you should never go cheap on your health. Spending money towards improving your health is not an expense, but rather an investment. Investing in the right people (Q3) and processes (Q4) to support you in maintaining and protecting your health is one of the most important investments that you can make. It is far cheaper to maintain your health than it is to recover it once it is lost. People know this and say things like, "An ounce of prevention is better than a pound of cure," but do they really practice what they preach? Saying something and knowing something are different then doing something. I have never regretted investing significant money in my health or personal development to make me a better individual, spouse, parent, physician, and community leader. I view investing in my health as a necessity just like a house to live in. In fact, you can replace a house or car, but you cannot replace your body. It's the only one given to you and you have to take care of it for your whole life. Don't go cheap here.

If you want to change the quality of your life very quickly, do this exercise. Think about all the people that significantly impact each area of your life. Now specifically, write down the names of the people that have influenced you in regards to your health. This list can include your spouse, children, friends, family, coworkers, doctors, and other healthcare providers that we've discussed. Write them all down. Then next to each name, put a positive sign or a minus sign, indicating if the person is a positive influence overall in supporting you in your health or a negative influence, dragging you down.

I have seen through the hundreds of people that have done this exercise that those who are *excelling* in a particular area of their life have significantly more *positive* signs next to the names of the people on this list. The people who are struggling in areas including their health, either have a very short list or a lot of negative signs next to the names.

The key then is to systematically eliminate the negative influencers and replace them with positive people, who will impact your life and get you closer to your vision, goals, and promises. The question often arises about not being able to fully eliminate all the negatives on your list because there are people, who, due to their relationship with you, have to be present. This may include family members, coworkers, or even clients. You can't exactly eliminate a family member nor do you have the authority to fire a coworker.

Here's what I recommend. Find ways to limit your exposure to these negative people. Again, this is your health, your greatest asset and it is worth protecting. You become who you surround yourself with, and if you continuously allow yourself to be surrounded by negative people, it will infect you. If it is family members that you do not live with, then limit your exposure to them to only major holidays or events. Make a pact with either your significant other or accountability partner that you are not going to let their negative influence affect you. Have a plan to handle these interactions intentionally. Keep conversations light and do not share with them your vision, goals, or accomplishments in the area that they are negative in. Don't try to convince them or change them. Accept them for where they are in their life and move on.

Now if somebody who is negative is trying to change, and they are in the season of doing that, by all means encourage them and pass on strategies that have been working for you. You can make a big impact. But if they are not ready to make the change for the better, then your encouragement will often come off as criticism, and they will defensively become more negative and attack what you are doing.

If it is people in your household, then there has to be some level of honest conversation and a mutual respect to honor each person's choices and how they want to focus on their health. Again, trying to change somebody who is not in the same season as you or is not willing to change can become very stressful. Instead, try focusing on areas where you can support and nurture each other while at the same time you seek out people who will encourage you, support you, and hold you accountable to your health goals and vision.

Synergy Action Steps

1. Who on your health team keeps you personally accountable to your health?
2. Who are the definite positive and negative influencers on your health? What changes to your team might you need to make?
3. Who do you personally support to help keep them accountable to their health goals?

Q3 PEOPLE—PEOPLE YOU SERVE AND CARE FOR

Everyone has his own specific vocation or mission in life; everyone must carry out a concrete assignment that demands fulfillment. Therein he cannot be replaced, nor can his life be repeated. Thus, everyone's task is unique as is his specific opportunity to implement it.

—Viktor Frankl

In the previous chapter, we talked about people on your team, specifically those on your health team. In this chapter, we discuss the people you serve and care for. These are the people who depend upon you in all the areas of your life. Starting with your inner circle, you have family and close friends. This small but powerful group really depends on you being present and showing up in a positive way.

Our children are a lot smarter than we think. They see us and mimic us. The things we say, the energy we bring, and how we carry ourselves serve as models for their future behavior. You are your children's role model in the crucial developing years of their lives. If you are unhealthy, fatigued, and stressed, then you are modeling that to your children. They will feel it, respond to it, and it will shape who they are. Our kids deserve the best version of us. As parents, we want to set them up for success. As role models to our children, though, rarely do we realize that setting them up for success occurs by setting our own health up for success. Just like how on an airplane, when the attendants are giving the emergency announcements, they always state if there is a decrease in cabin pressure to put the oxygen mask on ourselves first before putting the oxygen mask on our children—we cannot serve our children to the highest capacity if we ourselves are not healthy and are not willing to accept the responsibility to care for ourselves first.

Jim Rohn, an influential motivational speaker, said that you become the average of the top five people you spend the most amount of time with. Your close friends often have similar values, viewpoints, and interests as you. As part of the exercise in the previous chapter, I recommended that you write a positive or negative sign next to each person's name in regard to how they influence your health. *Here is where I ask the question in reverse*: if others close to you wrote your name on their list, would you have a positive or a negative sign next to your name? Just like your children, your close friends, who you have a profound impact on, deserve the best version of you. Like attracts like. If you want to have great relationships with great people, then you have to be great. You need to show up with great energy, health, and vitality, and add value and energy to the relationship.

Our spouses and significant others deserve our best. When I married my wife, I made a commitment to support her, love and honor her, and protect her. When we look at our wedding pictures and see the energy, health, and vitality radiating from us, do we still carry that spark and vitality today? Of course, we get older and our bodies change over the decades, but what is the rate of your health decay? Are you doing everything you can to be healthy for not only yourself but also for your spouse? Have you been letting yourself go because you have become all too comfortable in the relationship or other demands in your life knocked your health off track? Our spouses look to us to be the rocks in their lives. How much focus are you dedicating to your health in order to be a rock in their life?

Outside of your inner circle, what about the people that you serve and support, such as your employees, co-workers, or employers? What about the people who exchange money for the service, products, or value you provide them? In your line of work, your employees, managers, coworkers, employers, and customers deserve your best. I believe that the value you receive in the marketplace is based upon the value you provide to the marketplace. It is impossible for you to give the highest degree of value in the marketplace if you do not have strong health. Everybody loves being around a person who is positive, upbeat, high energy, and healthy. We like to be around them because they make us feel better. They lift us up and can potentially refocus our negative thought pattern into a positive one. We have all been around a professional salesperson who is positive and resourceful and who made our buying decision easier and pleasant. As customers in the marketplace, we want to be led by competent people who have our best interests in mind. If you are sick, stressed, fatigued, and in poor health, it will be very hard for you to be of ultimate service to others.

Before I was married, my main and ultimate purpose for maintaining my health was to be able to provide high energy, expert care to my patient base. As I've already shared in this book, I decided that my standard was to be able to give the last patient who came in at 6 pm at night the same focus, intent, and high energy as the person who came in at 6:45 am that same morning. And to do this for five days a week. You see, if it were just about me, I would eat foods that give me pleasure and exercise only when I feel internally motivated. When it is about providing high quality, impactful care that I know is critical to others' health, I step up and pursue consistent healthy activities so that I can be of service to others. The takeaway: allow your service to others to motivate you to pursue your best health practices.

Synergy Action Steps

1. Who would you say are the people you serve and support that require you to be healthy?
2. On a scale of one to ten, how committed are you to being healthy for the sake of the people that you serve and support?
3. What do you need to do that would increase your personal commitment to your health and the people you serve?
4. How will you know that you have increased your personal commitment? What will be the clear and compelling evidence of your shift?
5. Consider having me teach your team the elements of the Synergy Health Solution to create a culture that values and expresses workplace wellness. **Contact us through our website www.TheSynergyLife.com to inquire about our custom corporate Synergy talks.**

QUADRANT 4— PROCESS

The people in your life matter. You attract the people (Q3) in your life that tend to be consistent with your purpose (Q2), vision, and goals. There is merit in the adage, "Birds of a feather flock together." Your flock more than likely shares similar values and viewpoints as you do. The people in your life become the people you share life with. The people in your life are both teachers, students, and peers. The Synergy Success Cycle proposes that it is from the people in your life that you learn and adapt your processes, the fourth and final quadrant.

Our processes consist of the activities we do and the systems we use to make habits. But process is more than just the simple act of "doing." It involves the planning that occurs before the event. Importantly, the quality of our actions rises and falls according to the standards we hold them to. Therefore, the process quadrant (Q4) is broken down into these chapters:

- Chapter 17: Your Health Standards
- Chapter 18: The Work *On* Your Health
- Chapter 19: The Work *In* Your Health

The process quadrant completes the Synergy Success Cycle and fulfills the outer expression of your health potential. Like a butterfly that has progressed and grown through different lifecycles and experiences, the process quadrant is when, through your actions, you are finally set free to positively impact the world. Although process is the last quadrant in the cycle, it is also the one that initiates a new revolution of the cycle. Always bear in mind that the results you achieve are consistent and congruent with your current level in each of the synergy quadrants. As you gain new successes and new levels of health, then you are set free to re-evaluate your power (Q1) and begin a new journey.

CHAPTER 17

Q4 PROCESS—YOUR HEALTH STANDARDS

Be a yardstick of quality. Some people aren't used
to an environment where excellence is expected.

—Steve Jobs

The quality of your life and your health is based upon the quality of the standards you choose to execute in your life. When I refer to "standards," I mean your acceptable minimum level of behavior that you follow in your outward actions and behaviors, i.e., your processes. Your standards are on display with your mindset (Q1), your level of purpose (Q2), the people you associate with (Q3), and the quality of your planning and execution (Q4). Engaging with the Synergy Success Cycle will necessarily raise your personal standards. As you gain more clarity on your strengths and become more grounded with your values, then your belief in yourself (Q1) will increase and your standards will ride that wave too. When your purpose (Q2) elevates and expands, your vision and goals will transform. The level of performance you demand of yourself will rise. As you demand more of yourself, then the behaviors of those around you (Q3) must elevate or they must get out of the way. As you determine your focus, your standards for your processes (Q4)—both in planning and execution—will skyrocket.

Truth be told, we could weave in an examination of standards throughout this whole framework, but I mention it here in the process quadrant to remind you that your actions (Q4)—the outer expression of all this hard work you are doing to consciously elevate your health and your life—must be congruent with your personal standard. If your level of execution (Q4) does not match your standards, then you will not be satisfied and fulfilled with your results. Poor standards will only slow down the next revolution of the Synergy Success Cycle. Conversely, executing with high personal standards will propel you in raising your belief in yourself and your Q1 power!

Your health will increase the moment you make increased health your new standard. Clear standards set the "floor" or baseline of acceptable behaviors, so the moment you recognize that your actions fall below your chosen standard, you can use your standard as a springboard to get you quickly back to where you need and want to be. When you inevitably slip and regress, perhaps by indulging in some unhealthy behavior, your standards will offer you some temporary emotional pain. Short bursts of emotional pain are not a bad thing, but rather serve as an emotional cue that something needs to change. So long as you have your purpose (Q2) clear and the right people (Q3) to support you, then you will recover from the tailspin of a poor health choice and get back on the flight path to your MAGIC goals.

We all fall off the wagon when it comes to eating clean. We all slack on our exercise at some point. We all have been in a tailspin of negative limiting thought patterns. We all have covered up our pain in some way or another. To slip into unhealthy behavior is human. If it wasn't a continual battle to stay healthy, then there would be no need for this book! **In looking at this with a chiropractic lens, your standards are like your backbone that supports the posture of your life.** Standards lift you up, fight the tendencies of gravity, and strongly serve as the main part of the skeleton for all the areas to connect to.

If you don't intentionally raise your standards in the areas of your life that you want to improve, you will likely fall to the general standard of society. And when you look at the general standard of society, that bar unfortunately is not very high. It's very easy to compare yourself to someone who is less well off than you in a particular area. Temporarily this comparison can help you emotionally feel good, but in the long run, it can cause you to become complacent. Standards should not be set through comparison with others. Standards should be defined by comparing where you are to where you want to go based upon a predetermined level that you want to achieve. That's why you need to be around leaders in the areas you want to enhance. The people who are leaders, mentors, and coaches will assist you in raising your standards, but you still have to take ownership of your standards. You can borrow theirs as you build your skills, but you cannot become dependent on their standards in your life.

Standards Form Habits

Your standards will influence the actions (Q4) that you take on a consistent level. The actions you take consistently will create your habits. And your habits become your life. There's a lot of talk about habits and their formation. Some say habits occur by doing an activity consecutively over 21 days; others say it's closer to 60 days. I say when you decide to have a standard that says this is who you are and what you will accept, then your actions have to become consistent with your high standards. Those consistent actions will determine what habits you create. I care less about how many days you do something to form it as a habit, as I do about the emotional intensity you regularly apply into increasing your standard for that activity. Standards are the secret sauce.

High standards create high results. High standards create consistent results. High standards bring forth the creative mind to come up with solutions and actions that are consistent with those high standards. Look at any area of your life that you are doing very well at. You will see that your standard is very high. Humans have an inherent drive to be consistent with their thoughts, beliefs, and words. When your thoughts and beliefs are not consistent with your standards, you will deal with emotional turmoil and stress. Conversely, when you are acting consistently with your thoughts and beliefs, high quality actions (Q4) occur with more ease and will flow naturally.

Accordingly, if you simply decide to raise your standards in the area of your health, you will automatically see your health improve.

Our standards are also raised or lowered by the standards of our peer group (Q3). Because human beings are social beings that seek connection with one another, we tend to do activities that are consistent with our peer group. Smokers tend to hang out with smokers. Drinkers tend to hang out with drinkers. People who exercise and are into fitness tend to hang out with people who exercise and are into fitness. If you want to improve the standard of your life, you need to look at the standards of your peer group. This is one of the basic foundational principles that makes the Synergy Success Cycle work. As we become clear as to our purpose, vision, and goals, we tend to attract people that share the same standards. This reinforces our purpose, and through these people, we develop new standards for activities that we choose to do.

Raise your standards. Attach them to a compelling purpose. Publicly declare them, so now you have social pressure to be consistent with them. Engage with peers that share the same or an even higher standards. And do the activities required to get the results.

Sigmoid Curve

In business (and in life), there is a sigmoid curve[18] that explains cycles of where a company might be at any given moment.

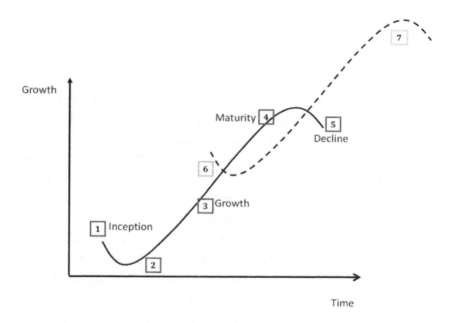

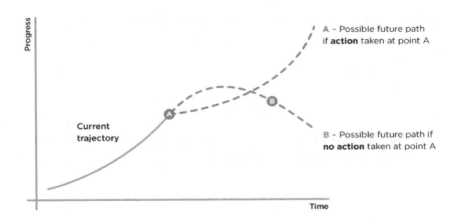

When a new concept is formed, it is at the inception stage. During this initial learning stage, there is typically a dip in outcome or production when the concept is first introduced. We are never all that good at producing predictable consistent results when we are in the learning stage. However, as the company learns the new concepts, they experience growth and move up the curve producing positive outcomes. This is an exciting time for a company as the rewards of the efforts pour in.

Once they get to a level of mastery or maturity, then results start to level off. Even though the growth is significantly higher than when the concept was first introduced, it does flatline at this level. If left unchecked, then complacency can set in, which marks a decline in growth and potential resources are needed to turn it around.

The problem with most organizations is that they wait until there is too much decline to make the decision to make a change (this is represented in the second illustration[19] as path B). This delay in making a decision to change focus or direction often occurs because the company is not measuring their growth, so they did not see the flatline and subsequent decline until it got steep enough or deep enough. The problem with making the decision to change at the point of decline is that morale is typically lower, and the financial resources needed to grow the company again may be depleted.

The key to creating sustainable, strong growth is to purposely reengineer a new sigmoid curve and start the process over. This is represented in the second illustration as path A. This is why we call it the Synergy Success *Cycle*. It is not just a one-time process but a framework meant to be repeated multiple times throughout your life and in all areas. The problem is most organizations wait to make changes until the dip, or steep decline in growth when they are pressed to make a change.

The solution is to engineer a new graph *not* in the decline stage or the maturity stage, but *rather* in the growth stage. This is represented in the first illustration in the new dotted-line sigmoid curve. This takes a very astute company to recognize where they are at and be willing to change things up even when things are going very well and growth is rapid.

How does this relate to your health? Most people wait until there is a significant decline in their health to implement any changes. Most enter the healthcare arena by actually entering the sick care arena because they now have their back against a wall dealing with a health crisis. In that crisis they have been depleting themselves of energy, sleep, and health vitality because they have been either ignoring an issue or pushing through it for months to years. Reacting to health issues too late in the curve will shift your health team from the players who value optimizing and maintaining health to the sick team players and their own set of tools and values. The sick team's tools often come with a boatload of potential side effects.

Examining this curve in relation to your health, most people do not see a decline because it often takes time, like the frog boiling in water comparison used earlier. Slowly and unknowingly, this decline down the health curve has affected their productivity not only in their work but also in their personal life. They have been slowly backing off of activities that they used to do and love. They are no longer exercising consistently. They are no longer having consistent meaningful interaction with their family and friends. They are covering up symptoms with medication, oftentimes for years without even much conscious thought. They are isolating themselves. They are getting depressed or anxious. Their fuse has gotten shorter with their loved ones. They are in decline.

Only then, when it is bad enough, do they go to the doctor. Again, the problem is the type of doctor they are going to and the kind of solution the doctor is going to offer. Can the person even put much thought into this because at this point, they are exhausted, in pain, scared, and just want it to go away? They put little thought into the care approach or how it aligns with their values. They are in a reactionary mode only looking to ease the crisis.

Now imagine if you made a decision to be healthy while you are still healthy, or even relatively healthy. Imagine that you know that this sigmoid curve exists not only in business but also in your health. Imagine if you accept that you want to start an activity and understand that initially you are going to put a lot of work in and produce little result. You're okay with that because that is the natural tendency of the sigmoid curve. Now imagine you stick through it and start getting some good results. This time instead of waiting until you become mature, complacent, and start to decline, you invest in getting your health to a new level by purposely reengineering a new curve in this area of your health while you are still relatively healthy. Now imagine that you do that consistently over several seasons of your life in several decades of your life. Would your life look better, worse, or the same compared to not having knowledge of this sigmoid curve and not taking the right action at the right time?

Synergy Action Steps

1. Identify where you presently are on the sigmoid curve of your health.
2. What makes you select that area on the curve at this point in your life?
3. Understanding this, what are some next steps you need to do?

CHAPTER 18

Q4 PROCESS—THE WORK ON YOUR HEALTH

Plan your work and work your plan.

—Napoleon Hill

The philosophy and approach of the Synergy Success Cycle proposes that you will learn best practices of systems and processes (Q4) from the people (Q3) in your life. This section on process is where the rubber really meets the road. This is where all of the foundational work comes together—from discovering your power (Q1), to recognizing and getting connected to your purpose (Q2), and attracting the right people (Q3) who will guide and mentor you to do the actual work required (Q4) to generate success in the areas of life you're focusing on, such as your health. Having a great potential in an area is a wonderful thing, but with no action to back it up, it has little value. In fact, I think it is worse to be able to know something very well and not do anything with that knowledge, especially if it can positively impact you and those around you.

Michael Gerber, author of *The E Myth*, states that we must not only work *in* our business but also work *on* our business. Many business owners and corporate leaders are so consumed with the day-to-day operations, that there is little reserved time, energy, and focus for making sure the company is strong and headed in the right direction. This is also true with our physical body and our health. Most people are so consumed by the daily demands of life, that they leave little time to actually evaluate, reflect, plan, and allocate adequate resources to ensure their body remains healthy. In other words, most do not spend enough energy on working on their body, mind, and spirit so they can really achieve their best life ever. By working with the Synergy Success Cycle you exclude yourself from this group and instead place yourself in a position of power.

Journey of Learning

The first step in creating an overarching framework for the actions you'll take to increase your health is to understand how you learn. I call this the journey of learning.[20]

In every area of life and in every activity you do you go through a similar journey of learning. The first stage is called "unconscious incompetence." This is where you are unaware that you are incompetent in a particular activity. Essentially, you don't even know that you don't even know. This is one of the greatest barriers to growth: not even having an awareness that growth is necessary or available in a particular area. So, the first step in really making a change in your aim of reaching your optimal health is to have awareness that there is so much about achieving optimal health that you do not know.

The moment that you reach awareness you shift to the second stage, which is where you become "consciously incompetent." This means that you become aware that you are not good at a particular activity and are incapable of producing a consistent positive result.

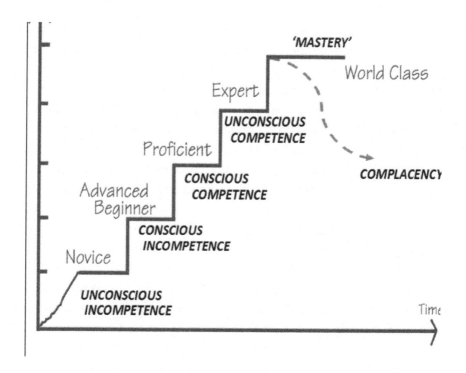

At this point people typically go in one of two directions. One choice is that they give up. Here is where your power (Q1) really kicks in. Your internal beliefs (Q1) about whether or not you think you can or can't learn an activity will cause you to engage or not engage. At this stage, people will look to their talents and strengths to assess their capacity to excel in the new activity. Additionally, your rules about learning also will dictate the amount of effort you will put into the process. If you can get past these barriers and push through the process, as well as the fear of not looking good while learning the new activity, then you can accept the challenge and move up, do the work, and travel towards the third stage.

Stage three is where you become "consciously competent." At this stage you are aware that you are good at producing a result but you have to put energy and intentional thought into performing the activity correctly. Between stage 2 and stage 3 is where a lot of learning and change occurs. Most people think that being aware that they're good at something is the summit; however, there is another level. The fourth step is when you become "unconsciously competent." This is when you no longer have to think about it to be able to do an activity and achieve a consistently positive result. This is mastery, and this is when an activity becomes second nature.

Looking at sports you can see a lot of examples of this journey of learning. Most people are unaware of how difficult golf can be if they've never played the game, which is stage 1, "unconscious incompetence." From the outside, it looks like all you do is hit a nonmoving ball towards a well-defined target. Once a new golfer steps on the course and tries to hit the ball, they become acutely aware of just how bad they are at it, stage 2, "conscious incompetence." For many golf becomes a lifelong sport that can be worked on and improved, which is why people who play tend to play it for decades, which brings us to stage 3, "conscious competence."

Golf legends like Tiger Woods don't need to consciously think about how they are going to approach and take a shot. Rather it is so ingrained in their nervous system that they can make all of the appropriate movements, without conscious thought, while making beautiful shots. That is stage 4, "unconscious competence."

There are so many more examples where people go through this journey of learning. For some it is pushing through negative thinking patterns. Most people who tend towards negative thought patterns are going through life not fully aware they are thinking and interacting with the world in this way. Many positive-oriented people can recognize a negative pattern in another person but choose to veer in a different direction because they do not want to be around a negative individual. (Remember, we tend to attract people who are similar to the way we are, as our inner work in Q1 and Q2 acts as a magnet to attract—and even repel—people in our lives.) Often, it is only when an individual "carefronts," confronts with care, and points out to someone their negative pattern or when a highly emotionally charged circumstance creates a teaching moment that the negative person becomes aware, i.e., conscious incompetence. After awareness, the person has to decide—do I want to change (and move through the pain of the growth through the journey of learning)? Or do I want to hold on to a potential victim mentality that has provided a strong level of certainty—albeit negative certainty—in my life? You see, people behave in certain patterns to meet their emotional needs. For the person in this pattern, they need to come to a fork in the road where they can make a shift to meeting their emotional needs in a more positive, constructive manner than their current approach.

We go through the same learning journey when we change how we eat. My wife went through a time period where she became attracted toward veganism. In doing so, she and I watched countless Netflix documentaries on the subject, which dramatically increased our awareness of the positive effects of drastically reducing animal products in our diets, positive effects for our health, energy, animal rights, and the environment. Once we became aware (conscious incompetence), then we went through the process of changing how we grocery shopped and what we selected at restaurants (conscious competence). But it first started with awareness, followed by a decision to make a lifestyle shift and move farther along the journey of learning.

When you can do an activity at the stage 4 level of unconscious competence, the activity flows. Have you ever been so involved in an activity you lost awareness of time as well as all the other distractions of life? Research calls that the flow state, a state we've mentioned already in chapter 6. People in the flow state are in step 4, "unconscious competence."

The challenge about being at stage 4, or mastery, is that over time complacency can occur. Complacency is defined as a feeling of contentment or self-satisfaction, often combined with a lack of awareness of pending trouble or controversy. The literal meaning of this word's Latin root is "very pleased." This is when you can get so caught up in your success that you stop focusing on the activities or principles that got you the result in the first place. We have all seen people at the top of their game only to see them lose their position by younger, hungrier people entering the stage. In life, you have to constantly be growing and learning in the areas that you want to not only master, but continue to master.

The antidote to complacency, which can occur during stage 4, is to literally create a new curve. This new curve is very much like the curve we spoke about regarding a new sigmoid curve. This means that the person who was a master at the current activity will have to go through the pain of learning an upgraded new learning curve in that area. No one likes to be very successful in an area only to see how bad they are at integrating a new activity. Not fun for the ego, but necessary for growth.

There are a few things to keep in mind. One thing is to realize that regarding everything you are doing in every area of your life you are somewhere on this journey of learning. The problem occurs when you pass internal judgment on yourself as you make steps on the journey. The judgment can cause frustration for some and doubt for others, which severely limits the rate of your growth. Also, comparison to others slows your growth and advancement. It's very easy to see the success that someone is achieving in a particular area without fully understanding the context of their journey. Remember the iceberg illusion we spoke about in chapter 5? Rest assured that people who are highly successful in an area and produce high results in that area are those that have worked very hard and encountered many peaks and valleys as they moved along their journey of learning. Again, realize that all of us are blessed with unique strengths and talents, which also affects how fast we can progress on this curve. The key is to stay the course and stay focused on progress.

The other key involves aligning yourself with the right people who have been there and done that, again the people quadrant (Q3) of the Synergy Success Cycle. These people can increase the pace of your advancement on the learning journey and help you avoid the pitfalls that commonly occur. Successful people have found "hacks" to move through the journey faster by aligning themselves with the right people who shared their processes.

The final key is to not resist the journey of learning but to embrace it. It exists. Don't fight learning and moving through the steps, but rather recognize the process and embrace it. It's far easier to swim with the current than against it.

Creating Capacity and Planning

I've been teaching time management and stress management for years. The simple facts have not changed. There are 24 hours in a day, 1,440 minutes, and 86,400 seconds in a day. Professional athletes, business icons, and busy parents all have the same time allocation. The key is how they create capacity in their life.

The dictionary defines "capacity" as "the amount that something can produce." Your capacity is going to be dependent upon all the elements described in our previous discussion on power (Q1). Your beliefs about your capacity in an area will dictate how much energy you will put in to create more margin and result in that area. Your health capacity is dictated by your power (Q1), your purpose (Q2) including your why, vision, goals and promises, and the people (Q3) who support you and share their strategies. It's always interesting that high-capacity people have the ability to keep adding things to their plate while consistently producing successful results. **High capacity is a mindset. High capacity is a vision. High-capacity people tend to surround themselves with other high-capacity people**. People who get results rapidly want to be around the same type of people.

So, if you want to increase your capacity in terms of your health, you have to look back at the Synergy Success Cycle and determine what is blocking you from achieving that.

Work-Life Balance

Work-life balance is a big buzzword these days. Most people want it, but I believe most look at it in a limiting way. Most people think of work-life balance in a non-synergy way using only addition and subtraction. They feel that if they add more work, then it takes away from other areas of their life that they really enjoy. Adding more work in this example is viewed as a negative. First, I would recommend to seek out work that is so fulfilling to you that is does not feel like work (recall the rule of 5/7 in chapter 11). Secondly, this addition or subtraction perspective is actually a limiting, non-synergisitc belief that will cause you to negatively approach producing more in a particular area, such as work. To exemplify what I mean: if you think that increasing your work capacity will negatively impact your life because it necessarily negatively affects your (limiting) perspective on work-life balance, then you will not put the energy and effort needed into increasing your capacity.

As you'll recall, the Synergy Success Cycle is one of multiplication—not addition or subtraction. It's a different path. Is it possible that you can increase your capacity at work, again producing more, while at the same time increasing your capacity in other areas of your life (i.e., synergistic multiplication)? What if you had a belief that it is possible?

Leveraging and Combining

Do what you do best. For those of us who are self-employed, the hardest part is that it feels like we have to do everything, work all aspects of our business: from answering the phone to cleaning the floor to working the particular service or product our business specializes in. The whole reason we became entrepreneurs is that we want control over our finances, time, and destiny. However, this control can also be what limits our capacity. Hiring team members to do aspects of our business—to answer the phone, clean the floors, etc.—is leveraging our time, so we can focus on what we do best and have others perform other vital activities to keep our business running and thriving. Leverage is an amazing tool that people vastly underutilize.

How does it apply to your health? If you wanted to improve your physical strength, you can use leverage to hire a trainer. To correct your posture, leverage a chiropractor. To improve your diet, leverage a nutritionist, meal services, and restaurants. If you want to have more of a connection with your family by spending more quality time with them, you could leverage a mother's helper, cleaning or lawn service, for example. That way on the weekend you are not cleaning the house or cutting the lawn and taking time away from your family. If you want to learn just about anything, you can leverage your journey of learning by studying people who have had success in that area. All of these are examples of how leveraging can help you improve some aspect of your health.

Combining is the art of doing several activities concurrently to help improve the overall results. Synergy means "even better together." Synergy is the combination of multiple activities that when combined produce a result that is greater than the individual activities. You can combine listening to a positive podcast or audiobook to your strategies for healthy living at the same time while exercising on an elliptical machine or treadmill. You can go for a walk, enjoy nature, and get some sun and vitamin D with your family, therefore, combining health, nature, and relationship-building. You can choose vacations that not only involve a break from the day-to-day but also involve physical activities. For example, compare going on a cruise where the primary activity is eating (i.e., over-eating!) and drinking versus going to an all-inclusive resort that offers sports, such as tennis or golf, as the primary activity.

Planning

Anybody that has produced a significant level of consistent results incorporated some level of planning. Some people have a negative viewpoint about planning because they feel like it lacks spontaneity and makes their life seem too rigid. The truth is that planning *creates* freedom because you can intentionally make space for the activities that you want to do. There's so much technology today, with online calendars and mobile devices, that allows us to really map out our day and life with intention.

In the past I used a paper date planner. It was so much more work than the technology that exists today. Any recurring event I had to rewrite, and any changes often had to be scratched out because everything was written in pen. Now with the advent of online technology, planning and using calendars is much easier.

I recommend the Google calendar because it syncs with all your devices and allows a lot of creative use. For example, using repeated activities. One mistake people make with their calendars is that they only put in unusual events that are essentially "add-ons" while neglecting to record their normal recurring activities. I believe your calendar should include even your regular recurring activities, such as your work schedule, lunch breaks, exercise times, meditation times, date nights, family activity time, and spiritual time at your place of worship. It is even important to put in the time you go to bed, as no one is forcing us adults to have a bedtime like when we were younger. We have to create a bedtime schedule otherwise distractions can keep us up for longer periods of time, like a Netflix series, which can ruin the next day.

I also recommend color-coding the activities based upon the different areas of your life that you are focusing on. For example, your work-life may be green because it produces green! I use purple for my health. I categorize blue for my family activities. I categorize orange for my personal development activities and so on. Find a system that works for you, but at the very least record all of your events, including recurring events, and color-code them.

The reason I recommend including recurring events, and color-coding them, is that it will give you an immediate visual overview of how you're spending your time so that you can see areas that you are neglecting and other areas that perhaps you are engaging with too frequently. Also, you'll be able to see where there are opportunities to incorporate other meaningful activities. I have found that when I slipped from keeping my calendar updated like this, the unallocated time in my calendar got filled by either distractions or the demands of life that happened to come across my desk versus the intentional activities that I felt would help take my life to the next level.

Momentum and Consistency

The hardest part about an activity is starting it. The energy that it takes to get a project or activity off the ground is harder and more difficult on many fronts. Emotionally—because of the journey of learning, we move from unconscious to conscious incompetence, and we become aware of just how poor we are at producing results in that particular area, which creates a lot of emotional resistance. Additionally, our skill set is poor, so we fumble around while trying to get results, which takes more time and effort. This is why there is an initial dip in results in the sigmoid curve we looked at in chapter 17.

Many activities feel like you're pushing a boulder up a mountain when you first start. It also feels like a tire stuck in the mud with the wheels spinning, and there's not much movement because there's little traction. Hang in there. Understand these variables, acknowledge them without judgment, become resourceful by utilizing the people around you (Q3), reengage with your purpose (Q2), and focus on your strengths (Q1) in order to get that momentum moving (Q4) in the direction you want.

Once things are moving it's important that you be consistent. When you ask most successful people in life who have produced long-term results how they did it, it often boils down to *persistence* and *consistency*. Persistence is intimately tied to the belief that the meaning of the work you are doing is worth it. Consistency is tied to your work ethic and standards.

I feel that it is harder for today's younger generation to put a value on persistence and consistency. Why? It is so easy to get access to information and get immediately gratified by results that it can oftentimes take seconds to occur. If I can learn something in a few seconds by a simple Google search or buy a product on Amazon literally at a stoplight, then how do I train my brain to build the emotional muscle to be persistent and consistent over decades?

You have to work harder now than ever before to fight the natural tendency for immediate gratification to get a result versus building the strength to weather the storms that will occur as you progress deeply in an area of your life. Again, I believe the first step is knowing that this tendency of immediate gratification exists in your life. Next, you must prevent yourself from judging when it creeps up because resisting the temptation for the quick fix causes some level of emotional pain. Then make a conscious decision that what you are working on has enough value and meaning that you will invest the extra time and energy over the long haul to make it work and produce a more meaningful lasting result.

Many aspiring future doctors do not enter the profession because they are fearful of the amount of study and coursework involved. Doctorate study is a game of persistence and consistency. Whenever I was studying and had a few brief moments when I wanted to give up, I remembered my mother telling me to "chip away at my David." She was referring to Michelangelo's statue of David which is made out of marble. The statute required constant chipping away by the artist to remove the unnecessary to be able to produce the masterpiece that lay inside that rock. Do the work and stay the course, and you will achieve your health goals!

The Right Amount of Action

This book is definitely more focused towards people with an achiever-type mindset. Most people who don't want to achieve more are not going to seek out books in the personal development or life development genre. The fact that you're holding this book tells me that you are a person who wants more for your life and for your health. Especially if you made it this far. Congratulations and well done to you. I hope this book has provided you value. But most people, however, fail to realize how much energy it takes to produce a high result. Again because of the culture that we live in, surrounded by technology that provides immediate gratification, most people do not understand the appropriate amount of action that is required to accomplish something big. Taking the right action involves first understanding that you're probably taking too little action and from there emotionally deciding and accepting that more action is necessary and then finally taking high degrees of action on a consistent basis.

If you want to go deep on taking action, then I recommend studying Grant Cardone's *The 10X Rule*, a book that I've mentioned already. To explain it a bit more, in this book Cardone encourages readers to take ten times the amount of action then they think necessary to be able to produce the results they want. Imagine if you want to improve an area of your health, so you create a plan to get there. Now imagine if that plan includes ten times more actions than you think are necessary to produce that result. You think that you will get a better result in that area of your health? There's no question.

I simply add to Cardone's concept that by using a synergistic model then you can achieve a ten times approach without having to sacrifice ten times the amount of time. It is similar to the results of Gail Matthews' goal-setting study we looked at in chapter 13. That study found that people who thought about their goals, recorded their goals, got connected with people to support them regularly, and mapped out a plan—essentially those people were doing a version of 10X to their goal setting—achieved significantly greater success than the participants who simply thought about a goal.

The key takeaway is to realize that you should be doing far more than you are currently doing if you really want a blast of change in optimizing your health, or in another area of your life you are looking to improve.

While this chapter has been about the mindset and planning behind the processes involved in producing results, the next chapter is about the work you actually do to produce the results.

Synergy Action Steps

1. How much negative judgment do you give yourself as you are going through and learning new ways to become healthier? How has that past judgment and self-criticism stopped you from achieving goals?
2. Who are some high-capacity people in your life? How can you apply their high-capacity traits in your own life to increase your health?
3. What are some health activities that you can combine that would dramatically increase your health?

4. Are you actively scheduling health activities in your calendar just like you would key appointments? If not, start now.

5. On a scale of one to ten, how would you rate the degree of action you are currently taking in obtaining your ultimate health potential? Looking at your MAGIC health goals from chapter 13, what actions do you need to take that are more consistent with the MAGIC goals?

CHAPTER 19

Q4 PROCESS—THE WORK IN YOUR HEALTH

*When you do nothing, you feel overwhelmed
and powerless. But when you get involved, you
feel the sense of hope and accomplishment that
comes from knowing you are working to make
things better.*

—Pauline R. Kezer, former Secretary
of the State of Connecticut

There's a lot of people talking about doing things to get
healthy, but until you actually do the work, you have not
completed the cycle of action (Q4). Cycles of action need to
be completed. We have to plan and prepare, as outlined in the previous chapter, but we also have to execute. We are human "beings,"
but we become who we are by digging in and doing the work until
we come to a point in the cycle where we shift to human "doings."
Nike said it best with the phrase, "Just do it." The Synergy Success

Cycle ensures that what you're doing is what you should be doing to produce the result you want.

Start, Stop, and Keep

It's not just about taking action, it's about taking the right action. In order to not just keep adding action steps to your life, which will ultimately overwhelm you and burn you out, you need to sift through your current activities to see what is working.

The following start, stop, and keep exercise helps to clarify this. When you look at activities in your health, you need to ask these three questions:

1. **What activities do you need to *start* doing to improve the quality of your health?**

Be specific when you write down the key activities that you know you should be doing but have not been doing.

2. **What activities do you need to *stop* doing?**

Where are you wasting your time? What is your method of distraction that you go to when you are stressed? Is it eating unhealthy snacks? Is it consuming a little bit too much alcohol? Is it binging on Netflix? Is it going on social media too much? Is it researching the next shiny object that is not really that important? What activities are preventing you from focusing on the things that are really important in your life?

3. **What activities should you definitely *keep* doing?**

I'm sure you're doing many helpful activities in the area of your health. What are the activities that you're already doing that you need to keep doing and probably need to keep doing consistently? Grant Cardone says, activities that are worth doing some of the time should be done all the time, and activities that you shouldn't be doing all the time probably shouldn't be done at all. Pretty black and white, according to Cardone. Recognize the activities that you need to keep on doing, commit to doing them consistently, and schedule them as recurring events on your calendar.

To help you consider the activities to start, stop, and keep in terms of your health, let's consider your health in a few areas by looking at the triad of health we discussed in chapter 3: the chemical, emotional, and physical aspects of your health.

The **chemical** aspect of your health:

1. What foods, nutrients, or supplements do you need to start taking today?
2. What foods, drugs, or chemicals do you need to stop taking today?
3. What foods, nutrients, or supplements do you need to continue taking on a consistent basis?

The **emotional** aspect of your health:

1. What activities do you need to start doing to improve your mental and emotional health?
2. What activities do you need to stop doing that are negatively impacting your mental and emotional health?
3. What activities do you already do that support your mental and emotional health that you need to continue doing on a consistent basis?

The **physical** aspect of your health:

1. What exercises, chiropractic adjustments, or activities do you need to start doing?
2. What physical activities, ergonomics, or exercises do you need to stop doing that are breaking down your structural health, including your spine and nervous system?
3. What activities that support your physical structure do you need to continue doing on a consistent basis?

When coming up with these action steps and the refinement of them, make sure that you are reviewing the other aspects of the Synergy Success Cycle to make sure that you are aligning with it from the start and continue pursuing activities that advance your power, purpose, and people.

Make sure you are setting up your health team and sharing with them your plan as well as having an accountability partner for each of these three aspects.

Go for it!

CHAPTER 20

SAFEGUARDING YOUR MOST PRECIOUS ASSET

The function of protecting and developing health must rank even above that of restoring it when it is impaired.

—Hippocrates

Your health is your most precious asset. Without its full expression, you cannot live out the full capacity of the life you were meant to manifest. You and those you care for deserve your best. This book's Synergy Success Cycle has supplied a framework for you to think about your health from a big-picture, whole-person, and whole-life perspective. It's not a short-sighted approach to health that simply lays down some rules about diet, exercise, sleep, and such, but an all-encompassing framework.

The Synergy Success Cycle's all-encompassing framework is founded on the premise that health is unique to the individual, to you. Achieving your optimal health starts with inner work in terms of your recognizing and embracing your power (Q1) and from there, identifying and fully engaging with your purpose (Q2) that is consistent and congruent with your personal power. That inner work directly feeds into your outer expression. When you have a highly developed sense of personal power and purpose, you manifest that by attracting and connecting with the right people (Q3) and doing the right things (i.e., processes, Q4) in a way that expands your health potential. This is the Synergy Success Cycle in action.

- The Inner Work
  - o Quadrant 1—Power
  - o Quadrant 2—Purpose
- The Outer Expression
  - o Quadrant 3—People
  - o Quadrant 4—Process

Whether you are doing so with intention, strategy, and purpose, whether you are pursuing a half-hearted "shotgun" approach, or whether you have taken a passive "I'll deal with it later" stance, you are establishing and charting the course of your health, both in the short and long run. On top of that, the same applies to your establishment of your power, purpose, people, and processes— whether you are purposeful, sporadic and half-hearted, or passive, these overarching areas of your inner and outer life are working in concert, influencing one another to allow you the level of health and overall quality of life you have today and will have in the future.

I point this out to show you that giving yourself the gift of a great life, via robust health, doesn't entail reinventing the wheel or starting from scratch. Why not? Because the Synergy Success Cycle's power, purpose, people, and processes are already at play in your life. What it does entail is harnessing these already-present elements with conviction and consistency so that they move in perfect concert with one another to positively and synergistically influence one another to create the targeted great outcomes that you decide for your health. The point is to remove passivity and/ or randomness from your method of addressing (or not addressing) your health and to intentionally engage with these elements that, due to their interconnected nature, will reap for you massive health gains via the multiplying effect of synergy.

The Synergy Cycle: Repeating and Expanding

When you fully commit to the Synergy Success Cycle, you'll be amazed at how much more it offers than you'd initially expect. For instance, it's incredibly motivating to work with the four quadrants and experience their multiplying effects, and next apply the enhanced you, that you become, to another (and another and another) revolution of the cycle.

As a cycle, it doesn't end with the processes of quadrant 4, but rather those processes produce positive results that when you revisit power (Q1), you have a greater sense of power, you've disproven limiting beliefs, and you have honed in on your talents. Accordingly, this allows you a bigger purpose (Q2), vision, and goals, so that you attract higher-capacity people (Q3) and learn and incorporate even better processes (Q4). Let me reiterate that the results you achieve will be congruent with your *current* level in each of the synergy quadrants. As you gain new successes and new levels of health, then you are set free to re-evaluate your power and begin a new journey.

Blind Spot Detection

Another significant aspect of the framework is that it helps you to discover your blind spots and also serves as a powerful tool to solve problems when you are stuck. When you are feeling stagnant, walk yourself through the framework to uncover where the stagnancy is located: is it a power, purpose, people, or process problem? From there, you can determine the solution with more speed and accuracy.

Break the Code of Other's Success

Finally, this framework helps you to crack the code of other successful people you admire and want to model. For instance, Steve Jobs had great people early on in his career. He partnered with Steve Wozniak, so together they were able to make greater progress by sharing their strengths. Bill Gates had a gigantic vision of having a computer on every desk and in every home. Martin Luther King Jr. had a compelling purpose and casted a vision for equal rights sparking a national movement. Roger Bannister broke the "impossible four-minute mile" in 1954 shattering limiting beliefs and opening the floodgates for other runners. You can understand their DNA of success through this framework. Related to this is the **Synergy Life podcast series** on which you can listen to interviews with the greats, interviews that will help you understand the greats' application of this framework, so you can learn and grow yourself from their insights.

For those seeking a more guided approach with the Synergy Success Cycle, please consider the **online courses** offered at Synergy Life University by visiting **www.TheSynergyLife.com.**

For those in the corporate world, consider sharing this information with your team to help them achieve their best health and life. Sharing processes is critical to growth and what could be better but to share the Synergy Process with your team? Visit **www. TheSynergyLife.com** to inquire about our **professional speaking topics and programs.**

Creating this book has been one of my deepest desires. I have been so blessed to have others in my life share these principles with me over the past 30 years. These principles were taught to me in various methods and pieces. Compiling them, discovering their interconnectedness, and creating a meaningful model has been my desire to save you, reader, from engaging in decades of decoding to unearth this universal framework.

Thank you for investing your time, focus, and energy in learning about the Synergy Health Solution. I am grateful for the opportunity to have spent this time with you, and I hope that you engage with me in the other avenues you find will help bring your health and life to the next level.

Here's to you unlocking your health potential!
Dr. Eric Janowitz

CAN YOU HELP?

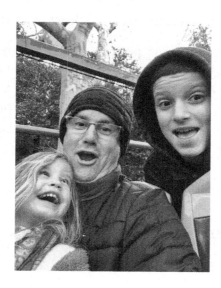

First of all, thank you for purchasing this book **The Synergy Health Solution**. I know you could have picked any number of books to read, but you selected this book and for that I am grateful.

I hope that it adds value and quality to your health and everyday life. If so, it would be great if you can share this book and help us get the word out about *The Synergy Health Solution*. There is so much information about health that it creates confusion, which results in people getting stuck in their health and, ultimately, stuck in their life.

The Synergy Success Cycle framework can help millions of health seekers, but they need to know it exists. Please help our movement to spread the synergy concept by leaving a heartfelt **review on Amazon**.

I want you to know that you are part of Q3 People in my life, so your review is important to me. Thank you in advance for helping spread the word on Amazon with your review!

Do You Have a Story to Share about How These Concepts Worked in Your Life?

We will be **launching our podcast** where we interview leaders and see how they have been using the Synergy Success Cycle in their life to help produce their results. We would love to hear your story to share on the podcast or on our website. Please contact us through our website at www.TheSynergyLife.com to share your synergy success.

For More Information on All of Our Products or Services, Visit:

www.TheSynergyLife.com

NOTES

1. "World Health Organization Assesses the World's Health Systems," World Health Organization, June 21, 2000, https://www.who.int/whr/2000/media_centre/press_release/en/.

2. "WHO Remains Firmly Committed to the Principles Set Out in the Preamble to the Constitution," World Health Organization, accessed January 26, 2020, https://www.who.int/about/who-we-are/constitution.

3. Peggy A. Thoits, "Stress, Coping, and Social Support Processes: Where Are We? What Next?" *Journal of Health and Social Behavior*, 35, Extra Issue: Forty Years of Medical Sociology: The State of the Art and Directions for the Future (1995): 53–79, doi: 10.2307/2626957.

4. George W. Brown and Tirrel Harris, *The Social Origins of Depression: A Study of Psychiatric Disorder in Women* (London: Tavistock; New York: Free Press, 1978).

5. *Stressful Life Events. Their Nature and Effects*, eds., B.S. Dohrenwend and B.P. Dohrenwend (New York: Wiley, 1974).

6. R. S. Lazarus and S. Folkman, *Stress, Appraisal, and Coping* (New York: Springer, 1984).

7. L. I. Pearlin, "The Sociological Study of Stress," *Journal of Health and Social Behavior* 30, no. 3 (1989): 241–256, https://doi.org/10.2307/2136956.

8. "The Most Important 5 Minutes of Your Life–The Wheel of Life," Coachilla, March 15, 2018, https://deals.weku.io/community-deals/@coinlibre/dicover-yuor-dissatisfaction-via-wheel-of-life-good-monday.

9. Ace Green, "The Iceberg Illusion: What People See Vs What They Don't," Medium, June 23, 2016, https://medium.com/@AceGreen1989/the-iceberg-illusion-what-people-see-vs-what-they-dont-see-d56dd464d5b.

10. *Autonomic Nervous System Poster*, 24 in. x 36 in., Parker University, https://share.parker.edu/autonomic-nervous-system-poster.

11. "What Are DISC Assessments and How Do They Work?" Assessments 24X7, accessed January 26, 2020, https://www.assessments24x7.com/what-is-disc.asp.

12. "What Are DISC Assessments and How Do They Work?" Assessments 24X7, accessed January 26, 2020.

13. "Core Values List," James Clear, accessed January 26, 2020, https://jamesclear.com/core-values.

14. Melvin Seeman, "Personal Control," MacArthur SES and Health Network Research, last modified April 2008, https://macses.ucsf.edu/research/psychosocial/control.php.

15. Christopher Peterson and Albert J. Stunkard, "Personal Control and Health Promotion," *Social Science and Medicine* 28, no. 8 (1989): 819–828, https://doi.org/10.1016/0277-9536(89)90111-1.

16. "Study Focuses on Strategies for Achieving Goals, Resolutions," Dominican University of California, accessed January 26, 2020, https://scholar.dominican.edu/cgi/viewcontent.cgi?article=1265&context=news-releases.

17. "Parkinson's law," Wikipedia, last modified on January 16, 2020, https://en.wikipedia.org/wiki/Parkinson%27s_law.

18. Marcus, Timson, "Defining a Second Curve: When Business Is Great, It's Time to Change," APDS Today, November 8, 2016, https://www.apdsp.org/defining-a-second-curve-when-business-is-great-it-s-time-to-/.

19. "Future-Proofing Your School: Do You Need Your Own 'Sigmoid Moment'?" The Key, February 26, 2015, https://thekeysupport.com/insights/2015/02/26/do-you-need-your-own-sigmoid-moment/.

20. Elisa Chavez, "Conscious Incompetence: The Enemy of Organizational Change," LinkedIn, December 1, 2015, https://companycommander.com/2019/02/18/4-levels-of-firefighter-skill-competence-a-fire-officers-guide/.

ABOUT THE AUTHOR

Dr. Eric Janowitz is an author, speaker, coach, and chiropractic physician with more than 20 years' experience.

True to the concept of synergy—he combines his degrees in psychology, human biology, and his doctorate in chiropractic to provide his patients with a comprehensive, holistic, and natural mind-body approach. In addition, Dr. Janowitz is a certified professional coach focusing on life, health, and executive coaching.

Dr. Janowitz has pioneered the revolutionary *Synergy Success Cycle*™ and developed *Even Better Together*™ programs that lead people into deeper levels of health and vitality. He is a passionate and gifted speaker who has fascinated audiences large and small.

To connect with Dr. Janowitz for your next event, go to

www.EricJanowitz.com.